CAREGIVING 101

Donna M. Trickett

CAREGIVING 101

1001 Easy-to-understand bits of Vital Information

written and illustrated by

DONNA M. TRICKETT

Library of Congress Control Number: 2011904176
ISBN: Hardcover   978-1-4568-8751-3
             Softcover   978-1-4568-8750-6
             Ebook   978-1-4568-8752-0

Disclaimer

This publication is designed to provide accurate and authoritative information in regard to the subject matter covered. It is sold with the understanding that the author and publisher are not engaged in rendering legal, accounting, or other professional service. If legal advice or other expert assistance is required, the services of a competent professional person should be sought.

All photographs of retirement facilities in this book have been printed with permission from the facility.

This book was printed in the United States of America.

To order additional copies of this book, contact:
Xlibris Corporation
1-888-795-4274
www.Xlibris.com
Orders@Xlibris.com
92621

CONTENTS

INTRODUCTION

Have you any idea what you would do if one of your parents or your spouse became seriously ill or had an accident and needed you to make monumental decisions for their health and finances?

Do they have a **will** or **trust** and a **living will** that is legally recognized in the state they're residing? Are you officially named **POA** (Power of Attorney) over both their **health** and **finances** or are you assuming that you'll automatically be in charge of all that stuff because you're their child or significant other?

Since adult children taking care of their senior parent is the most common caregiving experience, I will direct my comments to the adult child caregiver instead of the spouse or professional medical personnel, even though *all* caregivers of seniors will benefit from the information in this book.

First of all, it is important to realize that just being the adult child of your aging parent does not let you withdraw money from their account for a wheelchair or sell their house to pay for nursing home expenses. It takes some legal paperwork. The kind of paperwork that an **estate lawyer** can draw up for you.

Do you know what the duties of a **POA** and **executor** are and when you need to put each title into action? Do your parents have **Long Term Care Insurance?** Why do they need it and can they still get it at 78?

Then there's the question of where your parent should live? Should they remain in **their own home**, move into **your home**, your brother's home, a **retirement community**, a **nursing home**, or an **assisted living facility?** Do you know how **hospice** can help you and when to call them? Do you know how to talk in financial-ese, medical-lingo, and insurance-jargon so the professionals can understand you?

If these questions seem overwhelming to you and you're beginning to get cold feet, let me assure you that *Caregiving 101* will answer these questions and more, in a fun and easy-to-read style. I mean, if a retired elementary teacher, like myself, could get through the legal and medical issues with both my parents and even help other family members and friends who were dubbed POA over their parent, then I know I can help you. I didn't say I knew everything about caregiving but what you can't find in my book, I am confident you will find in my list of resource materials and from the help of the professionals that I refer to in this book.

The research for my book was based on my own personal experiences as well as the contributions of professionals in a variety of fields—and a lot of reading.

Caregiving 101 is not intended to substitute for any legal advice by the professionals; in fact just the opposite is true. My desire is to open your eyes to the many services these informed professionals can provide for you in your capacity as caregiver.

This book is also not intended to answer all the questions in a complicated multi-million dollar estate hassle but it will give you the basics for at least 75% of the families in America who are facing end-of-life issues with their parents.

Each state has different laws, each facility has different requirements and new legislation could change financial and medical benefits for seniors, so the need for informed up-to-date professional advice is imperative.

Why do you need my book? *Caregiving 101* is going to make you aware of which professionals your parent needs and what to ask them. It will help you be more informed of the choices available to your parent and in general make you a more confident caregiver.

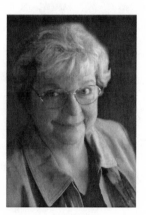

While your job as caregiver to your parent may seem insurmountable at times, it *is* doable. Millions have survived their responsibilities and many of those, like myself, have found it to be a healing and even inspirational experience.

So kick off your shoes, find your reading glasses, some index tabs and a highlighter and be ready to discover lots of helpful ideas, useful facts, personal anecdotes, along with a few chuckles.

If you'd like to share your opinions about any of my books, experiences with your aging parent or if your school, church or organization is interested in having our free *Caregiver's Workshop*, please check out my web page at **www. donnatrickett.com**

RECOGNITION

I want to especially thank my husband, Nelson Trickett, for his incredible patience, help, editing and perseverance throughout the writing of this book and his unwavering caregiving service to both my parents, Alice and Donald Killip.

On behalf of my husband and myself, I would also like to thank our son, Kirk, for all the times he has helped his grandparents and us, his personal heartfelt letters and the enormous assistance he has given to us in the midst of our computer glitches. Son, this book is for you when you officially become our POA and eventual executor of whatever is left of our estate. While the caregiving journey may be difficult at times, I know with God's help it will also be rewarding.

Finally, I want to extend my gratitude to the many friends and professionals who have given me their knowledgeable input, encouragement and patience with all my questions. And where would I be without the information highway of the internet that linked me up to the facts that I have recorded for your benefit?

IMPORTANT

Any suggestions given in *Caregiving 101* should not be used as legal, medical or financial advice. Instead, this book is intended to raise the right questions, be able to understand the professional jargon, find the appropriate people to give you the best answers and consider all the areas of caregiving that will help you to be informed, compassionate and confident.

I have consulted with professionals in various fields to give you a clear understanding of the terms and requirements of a POA and executor. Remember, rules and requirements change from year to year and state to state, so be sure to check all the facts and questions raised in my book with your parent's attorney, accountant, insurance agent, financial advisor and doctor.

Having been a caregiver, just like you, I have no personal preferences nor do I receive any financial benefits from any of these services. I'm merely offering you an unbiased look at all the possibilities.

AUTHOR'S NOTE

You will notice repeated references to several topics such as: **living wills, POA, executor** and **TOD** throughout this text. I have purposely chosen to do that because those topics bear repeating and some readers tend to skip around and miss a vital point. I'm hoping that the repetitions will help solidify the importance of these subjects as you become a more effective caregiver. Also, **bold printed topics** are defined in chapter 8, the Dictionary chapter.

CHAPTER 1

Understanding Your Situation

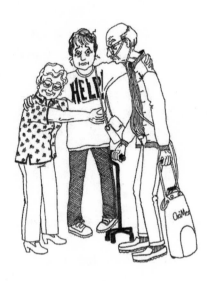

So you've been asked to take care of your aging parents. And even though you're not exactly sure what that entails, you've agreed. Well, congratulations! Join the millions of other caregivers who have stumbled into the murky waters of Caregiving 101.

You may be the *accountant-type caregiver* who figures all you have to do is pay your parent's bills on time and balance their checkbook once a month. Well, that's one part of it.

Or you may be the *compassionate-heart caregiver* who thinks that sympathizing with your parent's situation and visiting your mom and dad with little treats and warm hugs is the main reason your services were requested. That's good, too.

Maybe you're the *organizational caregiver* who can help your parent find the right place to live, arrange for all the right people to help them with their issues, and get them where they have to go. Lining up all their ducks *is* critical to their care.

Actually, all three traits are essential qualities for a caregiver of an aging parent. Oh yes, there is a fourth category of caregiving, the *clueless caregiver*. You just fell into the job because there wasn't anyone else able or willing to do it. You may be struggling with your own financial and organizational skills while experiencing increased nausea just contemplating the additional stress of running your parent's affairs.

Wherever you're coming from, welcome aboard! You're why I wrote *Caregiving 101.*

The calculating *accountant types* will be introduced to some of the emotional issues of their duties, while the *compassionate caregivers* will be shown some of the more serious responsibilities that must be accomplished. The *organizational individuals* will examine a few other issues they may have overlooked and be given helpful checklists to keep those duties in order. And as to the *clueless ones*, you're going to benefit the most. You'll not only help your parent get their golden years in order but you will be helping yourself plan for your own future.

My Caregiving Experience

In the beginning of 1993, I considered myself an ordinary homemaker. Well, I can't really say ordinary. In fact, I don't consider anyone ordinary. I think we all have unique talents that we just haven't tapped yet.

Nevertheless, my husband Nelson was still working at his career and our son, Kirk, had graduated college and was married. While we didn't have to worry about a strict budget, we still thought it was prudent to find ways to add to our income. Unfortunately the intermittent out-of-home businesses I began while Nelson was on the road, cost more to run then they earned.

In addition to my household chores, and running a faltering business, I was in charge of our checkbook. As a retired teacher, I had always enjoyed math and especially algebra but somehow algebra didn't help me balance the monthly statement to the penny. It wasn't uncommon to be off by $25 or $50. Usually, the deficit of one month was corrected by an unexplained gain in the next, so I always left an extra $100 in the account to cover any errors.

The organization of the cupboards, house and my time was sporadic. Our file cabinets were stuffed with papers and receipts but we didn't always know how to retrieve them when we needed something.

While Nelson's father had died four years earlier, his 79-year-old mother remained independent and healthy. And after triple-by-pass surgery, in 1987, my father was back on the highway in their Argosy camper. At 77, Dad seemed strong, stubborn, and sharp. He never asked for help in any of his money matters, not even at tax time. My 79-year-old mother was full of energy and able to care for my aging father. All I had to do, I thought, was make them happy by an occasional pop-in visit and family outing. Besides, I was the baby of the family. No one would really expect more than that of their youngest child, right?

Basically, Nelson and I had developed a decent routine. We visited our three independent parents about once every two months and had lots of time for ourselves. Time that we could spend enjoying a meal out, dropping in on our son and his wife, taking a weekend trip, going on a shopping spree or dabbling in a hobby. Within a few months, however, everything changed.

By October of 1993, my father's heart was failing. His doctor would put him in the hospital on Lasix to alleviate water retention and then send him home to rest with an oxygen bottle by his side. This treatment became so predictable that I was sure I detected a noticeable rut forming between my parent's home and the medical center. Since my mother never learned to drive, I had to set aside one day a week to check on Dad and help Mom get all her shopping done.

Not wanting to burden my brother and me in their aging issues, my parents had often spoken of moving into an "old age home"—their uninformed definition of today's retirement communities. While that was their plan, they hadn't actually investigated any senior facilities. Now, with my father's rapidly declining health, they were frightened about their uncertain future.

Nelson and I quickly began to visit some retirement communities near us. We found one that had some wonderful amenities and a nursing home right on the campus. If my father had to be confined to the nursing home, Mom would be able to walk to his room from her apartment. She wouldn't need a car.

As we all drove to the senior housing campus for an initial inspection, my father stopped by a bank to officially name me as their **POA** (Power of Attorney) over their finances. Me, the one who rarely balanced our own checkbook was going to be in charge of their finances. But what could I say to a father who was gasping for breath with plastic tubes up his nostrils? I said the inevitable "yes," and that afternoon they signed the papers for their new apartment.

That was the beginning of my responsibilities as their documented caregiver. I hadn't a clue what was ahead. I just took on each new task, one at a time.

Even though my father's reflexes were declining and his various medications had caused him to have two car wrecks within weeks of each other, my father fought to keep his driver's license.

Because he had moved to another state, he needed to be retested. I was sure he would fail the test and that would settle the argument. To my surprise, Dad passed both the written and the driving test with flying colors, so I threw up my hands in defeat as I gave him back the keys to his car.

To my relief, my husband took early retirement just as my parents were getting settled into their new surroundings. Thankfully, Nelson took over our own banking statements which gave me more time to think of the emotional and legal needs of my parents. Through it all, even though I was officially named their POA, my father remained in charge of their financial affairs.

After undergoing prostate surgery, Dad's health improved and he not only was back behind the wheel of his car but he got an adult tricycle and pedaled all over their new campus. Mom enjoyed the Jacuzzi, Dad enjoyed biking and once again I enjoyed my lack of responsibility.

Three years later, Dad was admitted to the on-campus nursing home because only 10% of his heart was functioning. Mom's legalistic keeper of their books was no longer able to handle all the details and was told he only had a few more weeks to live.

Thankfully, my very meticulous Dad had already hired a **financial advisor** and **accountant** and had gotten a **will, living will, POA over both their health and finances** and **DNR** papers in order. Mom and Dad both worked out the details of his **prepaid funeral**, right down to the person who would play "Amazing Grace" on the bagpipes. He also had cross-filed four file cabinets full of documents that would later test my analytical skills to the max. Dad could definitely be dubbed a dedicated melancholy-choleric (a seriously driven controller).

In his last days, he took comfort in knowing I had created a spreadsheet of his investment's anticipated growth that would provide for all my mother's future needs. Dad died in the nursing home and, because of the **prepaid funeral**, I only had to oversee the proceedings. It was emotional but not as taxing as it could have been.

Since Mom was never the detailed person that Dad was, and because she had no idea what to do as his appointed executor, I made the phone calls and mailed out the forms that got his benefits and policies shifted into her name. Once that was done, I made sure that mom's **will, living will, POA,** and **DNR** papers were in order and that all insurances and investments had the appropriate **TOD beneficiary clause** connected to them.

Soon after Dad died, Mom elected to design her own funeral. You had to know my mother to understand that it was more like a shopping spree in the casket room than a depressing experience. Her eyes were aglow as she selected the color of the satin to line her casket, the loving words she wanted embroidered on the pale blue satin, the roses she preferred to have draped over the top of the casket and even the hymns she wanted played during the services. Mind you my 83-year-old mother was perfectly healthy, but it's what she wanted to do.

Since Mom was still using her checkbook for shopping and she had balanced their monthly bank statements about 15 years earlier, before Dad took over, I thought I might just give her a refresher course in Checkbook-keeping 101 and let her enjoy her independence and new lifestyle. Plus it would free me up.

We converted Dad's office into a craft room and Mom seemed to be totally happy amongst her scraps of material and her good friends. However, when I began to discover unbalanced bank statements and strange stars and arrows in her checkbook, I realized that we would have to add her checkbook, bills and financial concerns to our own.

At first my mother resented having her checkbook taken away but eventually she gave in. Nelson added her bookkeeping to his weekly and monthly routine and I did the official phone calls.

That seemed to be working rather well until we noticed Mom exhibiting some subtle and not-so-subtle mental slippage. We came to discover that my 87-year-old mother was in the throes of **Alzheimer's**. Now I had a completely new area to get involved in; the medical needs and living facilities for a dementia patient.

Because **assisted living** and eventual **nursing home** rooms cost more than her apartment, I had to do some calculating to be sure I could protect her money for her future. Though I was only 58, at the time, I got educated in the areas of **Medicare** and **Medicaid** benefits while investigating the medical findings about this forgetful disease.

The decision to get Mom into assisted living was extremely emotional and time consuming for about a month. In the end, it was the best decision we could have made. (You can check out our personal experience with my Alzheimer's Mother, in my book, *Inside Mom's Mind*).

Mom still retained her independence and yet she was spared the fearful thoughts that had haunted her for months. *Did I leave the burner on? Did I take my medications? How do I get a nurse? What do I do with all this mail?* In her assisted living area, all those things were done for her. She could read, take walks, make pictures, feed the wild birds, visit her old friends and go on bus trips. Mom was delighted with her new space and once again I could relax.

Unfortunately, there is nothing surer than change. And so it was for my mother. Within eight months, she started to roam the halls at night. The next dreaded move was inevitable. She was assigned a room in the same nursing facility my father had been in for two months before he died. Sadly, with Alzheimer's patients, they can remain in a nursing home for years. While my mother was a gentle Alzheimer's patient, who was almost always grateful for the attention and services of her nurses and guests, it was still difficult to see her sleeping and mentally deteriorating from visit to visit.

We moved to Columbus, Ohio to be closer to our new grandson, but it put us three hours away from my mother. We could only visit her once a month. My mother's decline accelerated. She couldn't stand up by herself and her memory had faded into a torturous void.

After six months of long-distance caregiving, I decided to move my mother closer to us. It wasn't an easy decision because dementia patients don't like change and finding a vacant Alzheimer's room usually requires a long waiting period. God must have had a hand in the move because we were able to find a room and move her within two weeks.

The new nursing home facility was only ten minutes from our home. She would have a private room, about twice the size of the one she had. We put a bird and squirrel feeder in a tree outside her window and took her on little trips to the zoo and theater. Mom began to smile more as she surprised us by daily sprinting around the halls on her walker. Her previously despondent condition had changed greatly.

The new facility, next to her family, had improved my mother's outlook while increasing my responsibilities. I was in charge of ordering her medications from a discount provider, which meant I had to keep up on any changes in her prescriptions and deliver them to the nursing home before they ran out. If I didn't, the facility would have to order a month's supply from the local pharmacy which sometimes cost almost twice as much as the three-month supply from the pharmaceutical discount provider. With a simple chart, which you will find in chapter 14, I was able to keep her medication orders updated on my computer.

I always kept my brother informed about any hospital stays for my mother, changes in doctors and medications and the introduction of hospice. And I tried to arrange for regular family get-togethers with as many family members as were available.

My final act as **executor** of Mom's estate, in 2005, was to complete her desires for her funeral, be sure all bills and official papers were taken care of, distribute any remaining money and memorabilia to family members and mail out death certificates to the appropriate organizations.

While all my caregiving duties may seem like a lot of work, it was accomplished over a twelve-year period. In most instances, I had the time to learn and complete each new step before moving on to the next one. Paying bills, making important phone calls, keeping receipts, talking to medical personnel and adjusting to her forgetfulness became a part of our routine.

More importantly, despite some aggravating and even exhaustive moments, I found myself enriched by the services I was able to give to both my parents. Being a caregiver even tightened the family ties between my brother, his wife and me. How good is that?

Do You Know What Your Parent Is Thinking?

When you're all caught up with your midlife issues, you lose sight of what it would be like to be your parent. Since they may have a sizeable retirement investment and Social Security benefits, which you may not anticipate in your future, you may think they are well off. Truth is, like my father's $335 a month pension from the railroad, it really didn't go very far. And while Social Security and Medicare are a blessing, they don't cover all the expenses of growing old. For example; hearing aids, dentures and eyeglasses aren't covered by Medicare or Medicaid, although there are new Medicare insurances that cost a bit more but do offer some coverage in those areas. (*We'll get into those later, in chapters 5 and 6.*)

When your parent can't climb the stairs to their front door without being out of breath or experiencing sharp pains in their knees—they feel old. When your parent forgets to take their medications or can't remember what day it is—they feel older. They need help. They need you, but they may not be able to admit it. They may feel frightened by the things they've heard about nursing homes or greedy children. They may not want to burden you with their problems. After all, they're your parent, not your child.

Growing old can be humbling, defeating and a bit scary.

If someone told you that you couldn't drive your car anymore or that you'd have to sell your spacious home and get a one-room apartment, how would you feel? You'd probably defend your independence like a mother lioness defends her cubs. Is it any wonder your otherwise docile mother may become angry and stubbornly fight to keep her car keys or checkbook?

Your parent feels threatened by the thought of losing their old friends, their freedom, and the home that's filled with the memories of their children and grandchildren. Vacations, celebrations and laughter seem to be hidden in every fiber of the carpet and walls. Their empty nest is deafeningly quiet. Their career is over and the memory of their achievements is dim. Their vigorous health has faded and their future looks a little less than exciting.

Your parent probably wonders if they had accomplished everything they could have in their lifetime. They may wonder if there is time to fulfill their dreams or mend the broken bridges of past relationships. They are probably concerned about being a burden to their children or they may be worried about losing their independence.

A father who once held an important title or position often feels useless after his retirement. If he doesn't have a hobby or isn't particularly handy around the house, retirement may seem more like a prison sentence than a blessing. The more important his job was, the more useless his retirement may feel. Reminiscing is good, for a time, but finding something he likes to do is better. Help him to get busy in his place of worship, community or a club. Encourage him to take up a hobby. Woodworking, sewing, photography, art, or antiquing might prove to be fulfilling as well as profitable.

Women, who often feel their identity lies in an attractive youthful appearance, may be obsessed by hair coloring and face-lifts. Other women may feel their uniqueness lies in their baking and cooking. Since you've left home, they may no longer feel needed and even depressed. Sincere compliments about your mother's appearance, all she's done for you in the past or praises for the apple pie she made for you will go a long way to lift her spirits.

And like your dad, mom also needs a satisfying and rewarding activity. Encourage her to garden, make family quilts, help at the local school as a teacher's aide or storyteller, volunteer at the hospital, make scrapbooks for the family or write a book. That's what I chose to do.

Personal time shared together with your mom and dad is priceless. Of all the gifts you can buy, there is none more precious or needed than your time. Most reasonable parents remember how busy they were at your age. They don't expect you to be devoted to them. All they want is a friendly phone call or visit occasionally, which has no real purpose. Even a heartfelt letter or card with a note from you would be uplifting.

Yep, even your grouchy dad, who never seemed to listen to you when you were in grade school, is really interested now. And don't take grandpa's interest in your children as a rejection of you but rather as a way for him to make up for all the years when he was too busy to pitch a ball to you or listen to you chatter about the neat animals you saw at the zoo.

You know, another good thing you can do is throw in a couple of questions that sound like you're asking advice. After seventy or eighty years, your parents have learned a few things. Maybe much of what they learned was from their mistakes, but trust me, they know what they're talking about. And there's nothing like feeling needed and important again, especially when you're retired.

Try asking, "Say, Dad, could you tell me what to do for a plugged drain?" or "Mom, what did you put in your soup? I can't seem to get mine to taste the same." Now you may not really need their help but just asking can make them feel like a million dollars. They might even come over to fix your problem for you, so do be sure you have a problem or it could be embarrassing.

Another topic of concern to folks over 60 is death. Death is more real at 60, 70 and 80 than it is at 20, 30 or 40. Will it hurt? Will they be remembered after they're gone? Will their spouse be able to survive without them, mentally and financially? Even the most religious parent feels a certain apprehension when the ultimate truth is staring him in the face. They fear being alone when that invisible phantom, death, lurks ever closer. Take time to listen to them. Do they need spiritual counseling or is there some relationship they need to mend? *(Look over chapters 7 and 12)*

Do you remember what it was like to turn thirty? You no doubt noticed a definite difference from your previously fast metabolism, vitality and youth. Nevertheless, you were still able to play basketball, jog around the block, help your friend move, dance for hours, and in general, feel pretty good.

If you've made it to forty, you're probably researching wrinkle creams, exercise bikes and hair colorings.

By fifty, most of us have reduced our athletic participation to a brisk walk around the block and we may even consider a face-lift or hair replacements.

After sixty, the changes accelerate. Wrinkles deepen, muscles sag, hair gets thinner, and your energy fads into periodic afternoon naps. Few sixty-five plus seniors run the marathon, stay up for an all-nighter or plan another experience in moving via U-haul. Oops, am I giving away my age?

By the late seventies or early eighties, the sparkle may still be in your eyes but the energy and resilience has gone out of your body. Most seniors in this age group take several medications, are more susceptible to diseases and cannot handle stress like they did when they were young. Old men often weep more easily and old women are more subject to depression due to their empty nest and aging bodies.

Seniors frequently like to talk about the obituary column and their aches and pains. While it's true that many of their friends are dying and they probably do have arthritis in their joints, it's also a plea for your attention. Your parent is hoping that the subtle reminders of their reduced life expectancy and diminishing health will cause you to visit them more—out of sympathy. Mind you, they don't really want your sympathy and they also don't want you telling them they're old and they need to give up their car or their two-story home.

If that sounds manipulative and contradictory, think of seventy to eighty-plus-year-olds as senior teenagers. It's true, you know. We begin our lives as helpless babies in diapers, needing the care and comfort of our parents. Once our grade-school persona grows into a teenager, we start feeling independent and belligerent, but we are still in need of help. Most teens will tell you that they like to have their parent's approval and attention, not all the time but enough to know they're loved. And that's pretty much what your retired parent is looking for from you.

If you thought it was difficult handling a teenager, it can be even more challenging for the baby of the family to tell their aging parent what they need to be doing, especially when the advice reduces their standard of living, independence or personal enjoyment. So keep a sympathetic ear to your parent's point of view as you work out a plan for their future that takes into consideration their personal needs.

Money is another big issue. You'll probably find that your parent is excessively interested in the price of everything. Even with a decent-sized **portfolio**, they're probably afraid to spend money on vacations or eat out at a restaurant. With a fixed income, the unsteady investment market, inflation raising its ugly head every year, their increasing health problems, rising healthcare costs, decreasing health benefits, and the threat to Medicare and Social Security, can you appreciate their concern over money? It's more than a concern, it represents their very existence.

At thirty or forty, you most likely are in a good job or have the qualifications to get one. You're probably in good health and if you need more money, you have the option to work overtime or get a second job. At fifty, you may be at the peak of your career. But after sixty-five, if you want a raise in income, you'll be bagging groceries for the local grocery store, greeting people at the entrance to Wal-Mart or flipping burgers at McDonalds. The pay is minimal, the benefits are nil and with diabetes or just poor circulation, your legs feel like rotted tree stumps at the end of the day. Hey, I've done some waitressing and vending in my day. I know what it's like.

Even with a good yielding investment, ample savings, and other assets, your parent knows from past history that everything can change in an instant. The cost of food, a national crisis, medications, out-patient surgeries, hearing aids, dental surgery and nursing home care can greatly reduce their nest egg.

Can you understand why your parent may not be very excited about your purchase of a bigger house, a new car or a trip to Europe, even if it's something they enjoyed when they were younger? In the autumn of their life, they see it as a year's worth of groceries or medical co-pays.

Many seniors are asking, *where am I going to spend the last years of my life and how am I going to pay for them?*

Of course, some of you may be working with the *spend thrift parent* who feels they only have one life to live and they don't want to leave their hard-earned savings to their children. Having done without, in order to raise their family, your parent may feel they deserve some fun. New clothes, cruises and QVC shopping sprees may all be symptoms of their declaration of freedom, which is okay if their portfolio is large enough to cover those luxuries and still pay for future health needs. However, if your parent is acting irrationally, you may need to sit down with them and their **financial advisor**—and possibly their **doctor**—and honestly look at their mental condition and their retirement investments.

Don't be surprised if your parent feels frightened and often gets angry as their options begin to fall away. Your parent may think you don't love them because you haven't given them the opportunity to live in your home or they may complain that you don't visit enough. *(Chapter 13 addresses many guilt issues of the caregiver.)*

Your parents may think you're trying to get your hands on their money before they're dead and so they're reluctant to put you in charge as **POA**. A little heart to heart reassurance that you understand their position and that you will always discuss any financial moves with them, your siblings and the **financial consultant** before you make any big decisions, may help alleviate a lot of their concerns.

My husband, Nelson, and I have frequented several nursing homes. The consistent appeals we hear from many of the residents are, *don't leave me, don't forget me,* and of course the most popular one is, *I want to go home.* Often these unhappy remarks are because the patients rarely get visitors, they live in cold impersonal surroundings, and/or they have nothing to do. *(More about ways to make nursing home and assisted living accommodations more amicable in chapters 10 & 11)*

Of course, there are also the more healthy independent parents who don't seem to need anything. They may be able to get along very well, alone, in their own home. Just keep in mind that everyone needs love and visits and no one can stay healthy forever. When you do see their eyesight failing or their mind slipping, be ready to step in as their caregiver with all the official paperwork in order and your duties understood. *(More about what those official duties are in chapters 2 and 3)*

TRUE STORY

My mother-in-law was a healthy senior who lived by herself, by choice. In February, of her 91st year, she did all her own cooking and drove her own car. By March, things changed for the worse. She went from a bladder infection to heart failure in the course of two months. She died in May of that same year. I'm not telling you this as a prediction of the fate of your healthy parent but rather as a realization of just how quickly things can change.

MORAL: You'll be glad you did all the legal stuff while your parent was still able to work with you.

If you have to take your parent's car keys away, try to empathize and let them know that it isn't easy for you, either. Assure them that you'll drive them to the store and occasionally take them on a trip. And if that's not possible, make sure you provide them with some form of transportation so they don't feel stranded.

That's why retirement communities are becoming so popular. They bus their residents to stores and recreational areas, often right from the front door of their home. Their buses are wheelchair accessible and the facility has many activities right on their campus, from entertainment to shopping. (*More about that in chapter 9*)

If you do live near your parent and can pick your mom up to go shopping or take your dad to a doctor appointment, be sure to let them know it isn't a bother for you. Tell your folks that you look forward to spending the time with them or that you had other errands to run that took you in that direction anyway, so it isn't a problem.

In essence, do unto your parents, in their lonely aging years, as you would want your children to do to you, when you're retired and less active.

Thinking like a Caregiver

Whether your parents are sweet as honey or as grumpy as a bear fresh out of hibernation, whether they stayed married for fifty years or got divorced, they *were* your caregivers for a time. They probably changed your diapers and walked the floor with you when you were colicky. Maybe they gave you money for college or watched your children when you needed them. They may have even been caregivers to *their* parents.

I know this duty as caregiver probably comes at a very inopportune moment in your life, when you are loaded down with responsibilities and even some health issues of your own. Would you rather have strangers take care of your parent's personal needs? I don't mean the times that a nurse has to change their diaper or give them a bath; I'm talking about the emotional care that everyone is looking for. The kind of attention that only family can give.

Oh, I know you probably have some unpleasant stories to tell about the way your parent didn't give you the attention you needed after an injury or how they never listened to you when you were thrilled about scoring big time in a basketball game. They may have even yelled at you unjustly or been abusive. I'm sorry about that. But consider this: your children are watching and listening. What you do or don't do for your folks will probably come back to haunt you.

I guarantee you that being involved in your parent's care will help you to understand the aging process that you will have to face in the not-too-distant future. Hey, we all get old and we all eventually need help. This is your chance to show your children how to care for you in your senior moment.

I know you deserve a rest after getting your kids through their teen years, paying for college and working every day. Right? Right. And what about the vacations you wanted to have with your spouse or your grandchildren? Welcome to the *sandwiched generation*.

Caught between the needs of your adult children, grandchildren and parents, you begin to feel like a squashed slice of turkey under a mound of mustard, mayonnaise, tomatoes, and pickles.

The good news is that you can have your turkey sandwich and eat it too, at least some of the time. For instance, my husband and I would manage to take our grandson along with us on outings with my Alzheimer's mother. It was a win-win situation for all of us. Mom loved the outings, her 10-year-old great grandson enjoyed pushing his great grandmother's wheelchair and making her smile, and Nelson and I took pleasure in just watching them interact together. Joseph was learning how to work with an ailing senior and we were learning how to enjoy whatever moments God put before us.

Just because your parent is getting older and experiencing some problems doesn't mean that your life has to come to a halt. You can still travel, enjoy evenings out with your spouse and friends and relax watching your favorite TV show or read a book. Being a caregiver doesn't have to be all-consuming. Like everything else in life, you need to balance your time and remember that this won't last forever.

Look at your caregiving as an opportunity. No, seriously. It can be just what the doctor ordered for you and your parent. It may bring closure to the misunderstandings and hurts from your childhood and inspire a new appreciation for your parent's unique contribution to their community that you hadn't recognized before.

Your parents may not thank you, they may even shout at you or even forget who you are, but if you can still treat them with respect and kindness, you will feel a greater sense of self worth. And that's a feeling that you just can't put a price tag on.

Now that you understand your parent's situation a little better and you have an idea of what your job as caregiver will be, let's take a closer look at the specific things you can do to help them.

Also, if after reading this book you find you need further assistance in getting all the eldercare issues resolved, you may want to consider a professional **geriatric care manager**. This person may be particularly helpful if you're trying to care for your parent from a goodly distance; more about them and the other bold printed terms you have been encountering in chapter eight.

CHAPTER 2

LEGAL: Estate or Eldercare Law

(Discuss the following information with the estate attorney)

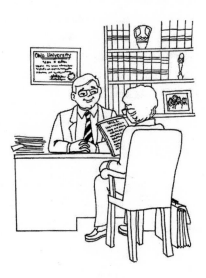

IMPORTANT

Encourage your parent to put together the following 5 legal documents and beneficiary clauses as soon as possible:
- **a Will or TRUST**
- **a Living Will**
- **Durable Power of Attorney over their finances**
- **Durable Power of Attorney over their health**
- **TOD clauses on financial documents.**

(All terms will be defined in chapter 8)

Aging is tough enough, but on top of all the health threats and senior living choices, there are legal considerations that need to be settled as early as possible, *before* your parent may be deemed incompetent or unconscious after a trauma or a stroke. No one likes to talk about **power of attorneys, wills, trusts, executors, living wills,** or **TOD** (transfer on death) clauses, but I do recommend that you deal with these 5 topics NOW, for both you and your parents.

It's a lot easier to cope with these serious topics *before* your parent is feeling physically threatened. And even if your parent is already in the throes of a serious illness or the beginning of dementia, it's not too late to set up some official paperwork that will eliminate a lot of court hassles and family disputes later.

A good way to get the legal ball rolling for your parent is to create your own legal documents. Sit down at your computer, with an official document-writing program*, or with an **estate lawyer,** also referred to as an Eldercare lawyer. You may have an attorney friend, but if he's not familiar with *estate law* and *end-of-life* issues, you are probably better off finding a "good" estate lawyer who should be able to cover all the necessary legal advice for a senior.

There are a variety of "self-made" legal document programs that may help you design your own legal papers. (Note chapter 15) However, they may not cover all the areas that are important to your parent or required by the state they reside in. These may be okay for starters but going through an estate lawyer can assure you that everything will be in order for your parent's specific needs.

CAUTION

As in all areas of professional services, you want to **be very careful who you pick.** We found some truly informed, fair and compassionate estate lawyers, some who only wanted to force my parents into expensive **trusts** and some who over-charged for their services. With the Baby Boomers becoming seniors, eldercare lawyers are popping up all over the place, so be vigilant. (More about how to choose the right lawyer in this chapter.)

TRUE STORY

*My husband and I never thought about wills or gravesites when we were in our thirties. Tragically, when I was 35, I was in a serious car accident. Our 5-year-old daughter died and I had to endure two months in the hospital. (The entire story is covered in my book, **Treasures from the***

Wreckage.) *My husband had to quickly purchase a burial plot, make funeral arrangement and, soon after my release from the hospital, we created a hastily drawn up will, which we later revised.*

MORAL: It's never too early to put together your end-of-life legal documents.

As an example to your folks, you can make up your own **will** or **trust** and a **living will**. Appoint a **POA** over your health and money, an **executor** for your will and a **legal guardian** for your children, if they're mentally or physically challenged or under eighteen.

You can always change these documents as conditions change in your life. Meanwhile, you'll be covered and your folks will see that this isn't about being old—it's about being prepared.

Since I'm not a **lawyer, doctor, nurse, insurance agent, accountant, banker, hospice worker, funeral home director, financial consultant**, or **religious counselor**, I strongly recommend you work with each one of these professional people on behalf of your parent.

Due to the variances in the laws of each state, ever-changing national laws that may be beneficial or detrimental to your parent and their heirs, you need the help of many knowledgeable counselors. Let's face it; the experts can make your duties easier. They know the ins and outs of all the end-of-life stuff and how to fill out all those legal forms. All you have to do is find the *right* people.

Yes, it will cost some money to hire these experts but a "good" lawyer and CPA can save money and hassles. You've probably noticed that I quote "good" several times. A "good" lawyer and CPA is the operative word here.

Any charges for visits with your parent's estate lawyer are considered expenses incurred as service to your parent, including long distance phone calls and gas expenses to drive to the attorney's office. Check with your parent's accountant and financial advisor, but legitimate expenses can be deducted from your parent's checking account if you're their **POA**. So, get your paperwork in order.

While some professionals, like financial advisors, give their advise free of charge after they are hired by you; most lawyers charge for office visits, for each official document and even for a short phone consultation. Most lawyers do not charge for the first visit. So ask what the charges are BEFORE beginning a phone conversation or even making an appointment.

Estate lawyer's fees vary greatly, as does his talent and honesty. Be sure you do your homework before committing to any of these individuals. If your parent has already been working with certain professionals, stick with them unless you have some very serious misgivings about their professionalism. Keeping the lawyer of your parent's choice makes your parent feel more empowered. Of course if your parent has to be moved to another location for health reasons, the feasibility of maintaining their attorney may be moot.

IMPORTANT

Get a portable ACCORDIAN FILE for all "copies" of the important papers you'll need to take from office to office. Keep the originals locked up.

Just look in the Yellow Pages, under *attorneys*, and you'll find a mountain of lawyers. And many more aren't even listed. You have trial lawyers, divorce lawyers, juvenile lawyers, malpractice lawyers . . . the list seems endless. If you look under **Probate Law**, you will find a list of attorneys who should be up on all the **eldercare** legal stuff needed for the necessary end-of-life documents. But don't just go by the listing in the Yellow Pages or a TV ad.

One of the wonderful things about having a "good" estate lawyer is that they act like a hand-held *legal Blackberry* before and after your parent dies. They will remind you of what official paperwork your parent will require. And when you call the estate lawyer to announce the death of your parent, they will help you through the official paperwork that will be needed to close the estate.

I've never regretted the cost of a "good" lawyer. A $100-$1000 legal fee to draw up all the necessary paperwork is not unreasonable and can be well worth the price, compared to the mess you can get yourself into without the documents. Prices will vary, depending on the complexity of the estate, the amount of time you spend with the lawyer and the state you live in. And if those figures seem too exorbitant, again, consider the documents that you can make up at home, that are available at office supply stores or the internet. *(Note chapter 15)*

How can you find a "good" Estate (eldercare) Lawyer?

- Ask friends who have used an estate lawyer for recommendations.
- Check the local bar association or the National Academy of Elder Law Attorneys. *(Check chapter 15)*

- Ask a trusted financial consultant, insurance agent, funeral home director, banker or accountant for recommendations. "Good" professionals often know other "good" professionals.
- Don't just trust an ad in the Yellow Pages or on TV, dig deeper.
- Be sure that the estate lawyer practices in the state that your parent resides, even though your parent may live just over the state line from the lawyer's office.
- Ask what the attorney charges for phone calls, visits and each needed document *before* hiring him. The first visit should be FREE.
- If your parent is an AARP member*, they can call the AARP Legal Service Network to locate a lawyer that practices in the state your parent resides.

Your parent can really benefit from an AARP membership. They only need to be 50 or over to be eligible and they pay only a small annual fee. They will receive discounts, benefits, informative AARP magazines and bulletins. Just call 1-800-947-9394 or contact www.aarp.org to get your parent signed up.

What does an Estate (eldercare) Lawyer do?

- Designate the **Durable Power of Attorney (POA) for Health** and the **Durable Power of Attorney (POA) for Finances** (first and second choices*). If both parents are living, consider first POA as spouse and then adult child.
- Draw up a **will** with assigned **executors** (first and second choices*) for the will or a **trust** and assigned **administrators** (first and second choices*) for the trust.
- Create a **living will**.
- Establish any necessary **guardianship** in the will for children or pets still in the care of your parent, if necessary.
- Create **guardianship papers** to care for a mentally incompetent parent, if <u>absolutely</u> necessary. (This is a very delicate issue, so approach it with caution and only as a last resort.)
- Discuss and create any other necessary papers under **Elder Law** issues, such as: disability planning, **Medicaid** planning, nursing home concerns, etc.

Two choices are made for these offices (executor, administrator, POA) in case the first person, presumably you, is not available for your parent when your parent needs you. Be sure second parties named in these documents are fully informed by the first named POA, so they can jump in at a moment's notice.

When is a Will *(last will and testament)* needed?

- Everyone should have at least a simple Will. Between husband and wife, it is often called a survivorship Will because everything goes to the survivor in the relationship. Be sure it is witnessed by at least 2 individuals (who are not listed as heirs in the Will). (If there is more than one page to the will, additional pages should be initialed or signed by your parent.)

  Also, understand that some states may not accept a handwritten Will or a Will drawn up in another state that your parent no longer resides in. That's why it's good to have an estate lawyer, to keep everything legal. You can always change the Will or even create a **trust**. The Will or trust with the most recent date will be the one that is acknowledged as valid at the time of your parent's death.

- A Will allows your parent to designate who gets what. If all their assets, investments and insurance policies have a **TOD** clause denoting beneficiaries for distribution of funds after the death of your parent, then your parent may not require a Will. (Once again, this is a good reason to have an estate lawyer to be sure your parent has everything in order.)

  Another thing to keep in mind is that you want to be sure that the beneficiaries have been changed if there have been any changes in the family status. *(Ex: If your parent was divorced and remarried, be sure the first spouse is not named as the primary beneficiary. Likewise, if another child has entered the family, through adoption or marriage, be sure they are named as one of the **contingent beneficiaries** in the TOD clause, or specifically removed, if your parent does not want them as a beneficiary. Once again, you need a lawyer.)*

- The Will may also allow your parent to designate who will be the **guardian** or **custodian** of their mentally challenged child or their fifteen-year-old Sheltie.

The more precisely the last will and testament or trust is written, the less likely it will be contested. And the less the family fights the more the family will heal. That's why it's good to have an estate lawyer draw it up.

As I mentioned before, you can create your own Will and living will off your computer or through services like Pre-Paid Legal *(Note chapter 15)*

If you are assigned the title of **POA**, check that all of your parents' valuable possessions: home, car, etc. include a **joint ownership** or **survivorship clause** so that the surviving spouse does not have to go through lawyers to get ownership of the house they shared for 35 years or the car that Mom needs to get to the store.

IMPORTANT

Make sure ALL deeds, titles, insurance policies, IRAs, 401Ks and investments have the appropriately named **Beneficiaries***.

Also called a **TOD or POD clause.*

(Simple definitions of these terms in chapter 8.)

TRUE STORY

My mother and father-in-law ran a store when they were younger and managed their conservative income very well. However, when my father-in-law died, no one realized that he had put the house and car in his name only. My mother-in-law had to seek the help of family and lawyers to get it all straightened out. It ate into her inheritance.

MORAL: Be sure you and your spouse as well as your parents have joint ownership or survivorship clauses noted in their deeds and titles.

Discourage your parents from writing any of their children out of the Will, unless they have serious probable cause. *(EX: If your brother is a drug addict and your dad is afraid he would blow his inheritance on illegal drugs, get arrested or die of an overdose, now that would be probable cause to write him out of the will. But if your parent simply wants to show favoritism because one child visited more or gave your parent more gifts, that's dangerous stuff.)* Let's face it, you'll probably outlive your parent and you'll still have your siblings to deal with, even if they're a thousand miles away.

Be sure that your parent has designated who they would want to be **guardian** over their child or pet that is still living at home and be sure that the proposed guardian is willing to take that responsibility.

If circumstances change in your family; a sibling dies, the primary beneficiary dies, a new grandchild is born, etc, the Will can always be rewritten. Or a cheaper option is a **codicil**. *(Definition of terms in chapter 8)*

Caution your parent about specifying an in-law as a **beneficiary** or **executor**. No matter how much your parent may love their daughter-in-law or son-in-law, yes it does happen occasionally that an in-law can be that important, it is best to not write them into the Will as an heir or appoint them executor. There may be some exceptions: such as a totally incompetent birth child or your parent has no surviving children or adult grandchildren.

And if the only legitimate heirs are grandchildren that are not yet 18, you may want to consider a **trust**. Once again, it's something to talk over with the estate lawyer.

While you may think that your family would never fight over an inheritance, think again. I have seen families that have gotten along just fine for years pounce unashamedly into feuds over who gets what. From houses to wedding bands, heirs can get ugly. So try to settle much of that through your carefully prepared end-of-life paperwork that you have created with the help of the estate lawyer.

Although it is possible that your parent may not even need a last will and testament because they don't own a house, car or business and all their remaining investments or insurance policies are designated with a **TOD clause**, it's still a good idea to have the legal document drawn up.

TRUE STORY

My husband and I had an elderly friend, Mary that we visited weekly. At 92, Mary shared her home with her mentally challenged 68-year-old daughter, Julie. When Mary moved to a two-bedroom apartment in a nursing home, Julie moved with her. Mary assumed her capable daughter would take care of Julie when she died but she hadn't discussed that fact with her daughter or written it into her Will. (By all means, don't let your parent designate a custodian without first checking if that person accepts the responsibility.) After Mary's death,

Julie did not live with her sister but continued living at the nursing home and found that they had work programs for her that helped her function in her limited world.

MORAL: Be sure that your parent states in their Will, how they want any child or pet, still in their home, to be cared for. They should name a specific guardian or facility that they prefer as the caregiver.

When is a Trust needed?

- If the value of your parent's **estate** (which is the accumulated worth of everything they own, not just cash) is $500,000 or more you *may* want a trust. (Some estate lawyers will tell you that you should have a trust no matter what the value of your estate—so you and your parent need to discuss this together and then decide what you want to do with the help of the estate lawyer.)
- If your parent owns a business or more than one home.
- If your parent wants total control over the way their money is distributed after their death.
- If your parent wants to designate money to one or more grandchildren for college, rather than have the entire inheritance going to their children (which is the normal distribution of the standard Will).
- If your parent doesn't feel good about the way one or more of their children is handling their own money and they want to dole out their inheritance in small increments instead of one lump sum.
- You may be able to avoid Federal taxes and probate with a trust, so talk to the estate lawyer.

Why do you need a Living Will?

- A Living Will is NOT the same as the last will and testament. The **Will** has to do with the distribution of your possessions after you die and a **living will** has to do with how you want to be treated if you are terminally ill or seriously injured and on life support.
- If your parent is ever unconscious or unable to speak, due to a stroke, surgery or an accident, the living will contains their wishes, as to how they want to exist. Do they want to be sustained by life support machines or not?

- Assure your parent that any important decisions about life support must meet the requirements of the doctor on their case. In fact, the decision to withdraw life-support is initiated by the attending physician, usually with the approval of a second physician and the consent of the POA over their health.

IMPORTANT

Everyone, 18 or over, needs a LIVING WILL

If your parent is ever in a serious medical situation and they can't speak for themselves, the **living will** is there to speak for them. One of your siblings or relatives may disagree vehemently with the possible need to stop any life support—but the POA, your parent's doctor and the **living will** document are all that really matters. Be sure that the living will is specific and says exactly what your parent feels. After that, if anything should happen, you can find peace in knowing that you're carrying out their wishes.

When is the POA over Health and Finances needed?

- Only when your parent is no longer able to handle their checkbook or their personal health care. Make sure the document distinguishes *limited* or *complete* power in these areas.

  *EX: Your Alzheimer's mom may need you, her **POA over her finances**, to sell her home and move into a nursing home facility. Your Dad may need his **POA over his finances** to only take over his checking account.*

- Even though the services of the POA may not be needed today, your parent should have officially assigned the POA positions as early as possible. The POA designated person or the extent of power granted in those papers can be changed at any time.

- Just being your parent's child doesn't give you the authority to get into your parent's bank account or make decisions about their health care. Only the officially designated **POA** has the authority to make it happen. **NOTE: POA duties END when your parent dies.**

The two areas of **POA** responsibilities (health and finances) are necessary to fully care for your aging parent. Even if your parent doesn't have much of an estate, there are always papers to file for pensions, social security, **Medicare** or **Medicaid** that require someone who has the authority to sign for your parent.

If your parent owns a home, however small, old, or under mortgage—you, as their POA, may have to sell it in order to give your parent better health care. You don't have the legal authority to do that as their child—but you do as their POA over their finances.

If the sale of your parent's home happens after their death, then the **executor**, NOT the POA, will be responsible for the sale and the distribution of the money; first to pay outstanding bills to creditors, the hospital and the nursing home and then to spread out the remainder of the inheritance according to the will.

TRUE STORY

> *I had a friend who was in a retirement community and was able to live comfortably and enjoy her senior years on her fixed income. Then tragedy struck when her son wound up in the hospital on life support and no one could find a **living will** to allow the doctors to "pull the plug" and give rest to her and her son, emotionally and financially. While she didn't go bankrupt, the stress was nearly unbearable.*

MORAL: All adults, 18 and over, should have a living will.
(I know I stated that fact earlier, but it bears repeating.)

Be sure that you maintain open communication with your parent about everything from the sentimental stuff to the more serious things. Discuss their favorite color, pictures and music. Find out what doctor they prefer and where they would like to go if they need nursing care. Be sure to find out about their medical history, family history and any medications they may be taking or may be allergic to. Ask about what programs they like on TV, if they're afraid of the dark, what they think happens after someone dies, their favorite foods, their pet peeve, and even how they would like to be remembered. *(Check out chapter 14)*

Also, if your parent is mentally or physically incapable, be sure the POA paperwork over your parent's finances, specifies power over **investments** as well as savings and checking accounts. If you need to liquidate a stock or rearrange an investment, you may find yourself powerless if the POA papers aren't specifically written to cover those areas.

IMPORTANT

POA papers, over finances, drawn up by the estate lawyer, do **NOT** necessarily apply to financial investment groups, IRS, insurance companies, pensions, Social Security and Medicare.

You may have to work out specific paperwork with each group or send a copy of your POA papers to each group.

As **POA over the health and finances** of your parent, you generally don't have anything to do until your parent's health begins to decline. Then you may be making phone calls, filing receipts, checking on medications, paying bills, filing taxes, checking on Medicare claims, as well as trying to make your parent happy. It sounds like a lot but it doesn't all happen in one day and you do find yourself learning how to get better organized, even if you never were before.

Remember, POAs don't get paid for their duties. POAs can claim gasoline, mileage, out-of-pocket purchases they make on behalf of their parent, long distance phone calls relevant to their parent's care, etc., but overall—it's a labor of love. (Be sure to keep receipts for any of those legitimate claims.)

If your parent wishes to reward you in some way, and it isn't jeopardizing their health or lifestyle, they may want to give you the legal allowable **gift** from their investments. (Check with their financial consultant, estate lawyer, your parent's doctor and living facility to be sure you are calculating their situation properly. Also, it's best to be sure that any gifting is equally distributed to all heirs to avoid family feuds later.) If gifting large sums of money is out of the question, your parent may choose to offer to take you out to dinner, go on a trip together or make you a homemade pumpkin pie. While it's not necessary, little perks do help to make the long wade through phone prompts and hold music for tax and medical information or extensive waits in a doctor's office a little more tolerable, so enjoy whatever gifts your parent offers, *guilt free*.

Usually a parent feels more comfortable when they have given something for all your work. So don't turn down any sized gift, even if it's brownies and you're on a diet.

While your POA duties will have some critical days when your life comes to an abrupt halt, these moments are normally short-lived. Monthly bill paying, an occasional trip to the doctor and regular visits to your parent's home become the normal routine.

What are the Executor's duties?

- Immediately after the death of your parent, your duty as **executor** begins. (The executor is named in the will.) If the executor is **not** you but you are POA over their money, be sure to inform the executor about any bills, discussions with your parent over their funeral or distribution of memorabilia not mentioned in the Will and the phone numbers and addresses of all the important persons that need to be informed*. (Note chapter 14)
- To execute or carry out the wishes of the Will.
- To be sure all bills are paid.* Careful! Don't be in a rush to assume you've settled your parent's estate. It's amazing how long it takes for all the doctor and hospital bills to roll in after they've run them through the insurance companies. It may take six months to a year.
- To submit a tax statement regarding the amount of the estate. This is where your estate lawyer can help you file the statement and determine if any taxes are due, according to the size of your parent's estate and the rules of the state they died in. (Check with the estate lawyer, to be sure you haven't missed anything.)

* The above is why it's a good idea to have your parent consider making their POA and executor the same person. And consider setting up the POA as a joint account with your parent's checking and savings. It will allow you, the POA, to quickly pay bills or purchase medical equipment, while your parent is still alive. It will also grant you, the executor, to quickly settle outstanding bills so that you can close the estate. It's a lot of power but there are laws against the abuse of that power, so be a good steward or you could wind up in court.

IMPORTANT

You are only POA as long as your parent is alive.
AFTER your parent's death,
POA duties END and the **Executor duties begin**.

So that no one in your family feels uncomfortable with you in charge of so much power over your parent's health and finances, be sure to institute family consultations (over the phone or in person). That way all the children interested in your parent's welfare can be informed as to your parent's problems, needs and use of their finances.

Keeping everyone informed can dissolve a lot of suspicions and solidify your relationships with your siblings. It may also reduce ongoing family feuds and allow your siblings to better understand the work involved in being POA for your parent.

TRUE STORY

I called my brother any time our mother was ill or there was a change in her financial status. He probably felt a bit pestered at times but he was always aware of what I was doing and why I was doing it. Bill and I have outlived our parents and we are still able to enjoy conversations together.

MORAL: Keep up communications with your family, especially with your brothers and sisters.

Also, if anything should happen to you, these family consultations will keep the secondary POA informed of any recent issues and be able to take up where you left off. If both parents are alive and one dies, the surviving parent is normally named the executor of the Will. It really isn't until after the death of the second parent that your duties will be required as **executor**.

However, if your parent, who is appointed executor in their spouse's will, is not well or able to handle official issues, you may find yourself doing all the duties of executor for them while they simply sign the papers. So be ready to serve in that capacity, if necessary.

In the case of my 83 year-old mother, after my father died, I unofficially took over her duties by making all the necessary phone calls and writing all the letters to Social Security, the Railroad Pension Board, and others. Mom simply signed the official papers and wrote letters to all the friends that called and offered their condolences. So it doesn't hurt to be familiar with the duties of an executor even before you have to be one.

The Survivorship and Beneficiaries chart on the following page will simplify how the normal distribution of an estate is designated in the Will.

Survivorships & Beneficiaries

Most wills show the inheritance going to the survivor...hence it's called a **survivorship will**, which should also include secondary beneficiaries, like the children.

As a caregiver, be sure your parent's will is in order with appropriate survivorship or beneficiary clauses.

Statistically speaking, women outlive men, therefore, I am showing the husband's inheritance going to the wife.

Surviving spouse should be sure their will is updated and expressly lists all heirs (their children) as their beneficiaries.

PARENTS of You and Your Spouse

YOU and Your Spouse

Surviving spouse would normally will their inheritance to surviving children as PRIMARY beneficiaries.

If Children are deceased,

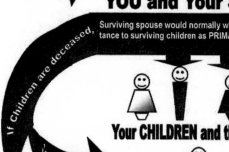

Normally the heirs are only your own children rather than their spouses.

Your CHILDREN and their spouses

Secondary Beneficiaries

Grandchildren can be primary beneficiary along with your children, especially if there is only one child or the grandchild is completing college.

Your Grandchildren

Secondary Beneficiaries

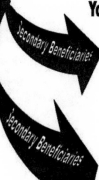

Non-Profit Organizations

Often a percentage of an inheritance is left to a church, research, or other good cause.

IMPORTANT

In regards to the following papers: **Will** or **Trust, Living Will, DNR, POA over health,** and **POA over finances,** you should have copies or originals of them in the following places . . .

Have an **ORIGINAL** of the above documents in:

- A safe place in YOUR home
- A safe place in your PARENT'S home
- In the possession of the second POA
- In your parent's estate lawyer's file

Have **COPIES** of the Living Will and DNR papers in the hands of health providers of your parent:

- Hospital (even for a short stay)
- Nursing Home
- Assisted Living Facility
- Parent's Doctor
- Nurses' station in retirement facility
- and Your accordion file

Be sure your parent's living spouse (not x-spouse) is named PRIMARY POA in both POA papers for each of your parents in case one parent is incapacitated when important transactions need to be made like selling a house or car that is in both of their names.

When the duties of the **executor** of the Will begins, the executor will need to know who to call after their parent dies; funeral home, relatives, social security office, pension office, banks, investment agencies, etc. (*Note chapter 14*)

CHAPTER 3

FINANCIAL:
Financial Advisor, CPA, Banker

(Discuss the following information with the financial professionals)

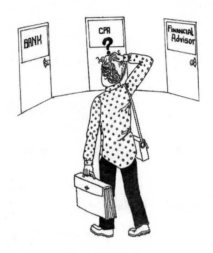

Financial Advisor

Many **financial advisors**, also called **financial planners** or **financial consultants,** will offer free meals before or after a lecture on financial planning as an introduction to their services. Your only obligation is to sit through the meeting and you may be asked to sign up for a personal "free" consultation about your parent's financial situation. Hey, a free meal isn't such a bad way for you and your parent to get to know their perspective consultant.

When you are meeting with a Financial Planner . . .

- Don't be afraid to ask lots of questions.
  (*To be able to speak and understand the language of the financial experts, look over the Financial and Insurance section in chapter 8.*)

- Evaluate how you and your parent feel about the financial consultant.
  - Does he/she seem honest and knowledgeable?
  - Does he/she answer your questions?
  - Do you both feel comfortable with him/her?

- Always be skeptical of "get-rich-quick" proposals.

- Check how long the consultant, their company and the investment portfolio they are proposing have been around. Has the company and fund existed and done reasonably well since 1980?

- As with all advisors, pick them wisely. Don't just choose an advisor because you are friends. Ask around.

- The Securities and Exchange Commission warns about any agents with the titles "senior specialist" or "senior counselor" which may indicate that they do not have the proper credentials to sell investments and insurance. Check out: **www.sec.gov/investor/ brokers.htm**

- Use your parent's financial planner as a consultant, not the final word. You need to learn a little about the market and what's going on with your parent's funds and other investments as well as your parent's willingness to take some risk. You should be able to have free consultations and ask questions whenever you have concerns. But don't overuse this privilege. Remember, your consultant has other clients and a personal life.

A good financial consultant should be able to guide you towards the right strategy to work your parent's money in a way that will best preserve it, provide income and hopefully increase it.

Remember, a financial consultant can NOT see into the future. They can NOT guarantee that your parent's investments will grow or that they won't lose money, short term. That's why you want to check that your parent's portfolio isn't filled with high risk investments. Ask to see other investment options and what you can expect from them.

Like everything else, there are knowledgeable consultants, not so good ones and very poor ones. So don't just go by the Yellow Pages, their credentials on the wall or the name of their company that you've seen on TV. Check the history of the **mutual fund** and the investment company your parent may be considering.

Your parent's advisor should be able to tell you how they get paid for their services and give you twenty year historical numbers of your parent's suggested **portfolio**. While there is no guarantee that it will do as well as it did twenty years ago, it should give you an idea of what it *can* do if the market is able to respond the way it has over the past. Again, you want to be sure that this financial advisor is being reasonably conservative and diversified with your parent's money because your folks aren't young enough to recuperate any major losses in a risky investment.

If your parent already has a financial advisor but your parent needs to move to a new residence that may be in another state, it may be a good idea to give notice to the old advisor and find a new advisor with the same company in your parent's new location.

You may be surprised to what lengths an advisor will go to keep their client. We have found that long distance consulting, especially over state lines, can be more expensive and less effective because of differences in state laws and lack of accessibility to the agent when you need them. However, if you find that the advisor has been excellent, it is possible to maintain the same advisor, even if it is by long distance.

If at all possible, be sure you allow your parent to be involved in the selection process and any financial decisions. While a number of parents are perfectly happy to let someone else take care of all their financial matters, others may demand to be involved in everything.

So that you don't raise ethical concerns, it may be best not to hire the same person that you are using as a financial consultant, accountant or lawyer, even though it makes it easier for you. Other family members may feel you are trying to balance the scales in your favor. While you may be confident about the company that you have chosen, at least consider selecting another consultant or agent within that company for your parent's affairs. Or at least talk it over with the rest of the family. Building bridges and keeping peace in the family should be a critical concern. On the other hand, if siblings tend to feud no matter what you do, you need to remember that your main allegiance is to your parent. As POA, your mom and dad need to trust you emphatically.

If your parent's estate is quite sizable according to your parent's financial advisor, not just *your* opinion, you may want to talk to your parent and their financial advisor about *gifting* to the heirs.

Gifting is a legal means of protecting your parent's estate from exorbitant inheritance taxes after they die. Gifting can also be gratifying for your parent.

They can watch their money going to good use, while they're still alive. The gifted money may go towards a grandchild's education, a family trip together or the down payment for a new home for one of their children.

Careful you don't sound like a greedy heir who wants your parent's money—now! How did you feel when your teenager only did their chores or spoke sweetly to you because they wanted some money to go to the movies? Well, maybe it's not exactly the same thing but you get the picture.

There are rules that need to be followed when gifting and you want to be careful that the gifts do not jeopardize your parent's future care. Your parent's $500,000 IRA may seem like a lot of money to you when you're only earning about $50,000 a year but if that's all the investment or income your 65-year-old parent has to last their lifetime (which could be another 30 years), that leaves them a little over $16,000 to live off of annually. Even with Social Security income, they are well below poverty level. So listen to the "trusted" financial consultant and accountant before going forward in the area of gifting.

Gifting must be done within specified limitations and it's best if it is done equally to all the heirs. Remember, it will be taxable to your parent if it's being withdrawn from their tax-deferred investment. That's where an accountant comes in. Run your thoughts through your parent's **accountant** and their **financial planner's** calculator and see if they agree. And if your parent is still rather young and healthy, you may want to postpone any gifting. Alzheimer's symptoms often don't appear until after age 85, and then your parent may require eight or more years in a nursing home facility. So be careful with their money.

And don't think you can gift your parent's assets down to the low-income or poverty level and have **Medicaid** take care of them. New laws allow Medicaid to look back five years or more to see if your parent had adequate funds that may have *mysteriously* disappeared. And if you were assisting your parent, as POA over their finances and gifting, you may find *yourself* in legal trouble.

IMPORTANT

If there are **annuities**, **stocks** or **bonds** under separate accounts—work with your parent's financial advisor to get them all listed together—under **ONE account**. It will make it easier to deal with after the death of your parent.

Have ALL the investments designated with a **TOD** (Transfer On Death clause). That way all the investments will automatically be equally divided between your parent's heirs. Each brother or sister can opt to hang onto the investment or cash it in. The choice is theirs.

Be aware that you may have to pay taxes on the inheritance—so don't spend it all until all creditors and doctors are paid, which could take 6 months to a year. And check with *your* estate lawyer, financial consultant and accountant, when you do accept an inheritance to see how it will affect *your* annual income.

If you've never invested or talked the "financial jargon" before, I recommend you check over *chapter 8*, so you can be a bit more conversant on the subject. And if you want a delightfully illustrated and informative book on finances that I have enjoyed, try reading **The Wall Street Journal's Guide to Understanding Personal Finance** by Kenneth Morris and Alan Siegel, listed in *chapter 15*. Trust me. It's a full-color book, filled with fun charts and graphs and actually quite easy to understand.

IMPORTANT

Just as another reminder, because it's very important that your parent has **TOD clauses** on all financial assets (CDs, Mutual Funds, and Investments in your parent's portfolio). *(Note chapter 8 for definitions)*

CPA (Certified Public Accountant) or Accountant

While you can do your parent's taxes yourself, an accountant or CPA is a wonderful addition to your parent's advisors. He can save you hundreds of dollars because he's aware of the latest tax laws that benefit seniors under **Social Security** or **Medicare**; laws you may not be aware of. And he's especially important when your parents are in business for themselves. Not only that but it's less nerve racking for you on April 15th.

If your parent's finances will allow and if you are POA over their finances, you may want to hire an accountant to take care of the tax returns and even the monthly bank statements. However, if you're thinking of putting a "stranger" in charge of your parent's entire estate and paying exorbitant prices for their services, you may want to think that one through more thoroughly.

As in the case of the estate lawyer, do check the anticipated costs of their services before actually hiring them. CPA fees can vary greatly, especially if your parent has a complex estate with individual investments, houses, bank accounts and medical expenses. Also, like the estate lawyer, be sure to ask what they charge for appointments and phone consultations before you begin using their services. Most CPAs only charge for their services, not hourly rates or for each phone consultation. I've found that a good accountant will pay for himself in the financial benefits they are able to locate for your parent—and they keep you legal.

Banker

As POA of your parent's finances, it may benefit you to set up your parent's checking and savings as a **joint account** with you noted as POA, especially since your parent might eventually suffer from dementia or a stroke. This will give you the ability to sign checks for immediate needs. Also, after their death, the joint owner of the account, *that's you*, will have charge over the money to pay outstanding bills from the estate even if the will is still tied up in probate. If you are not the executor of the will, be sure to make the money in the account available to the executor to close the estate.

If you are having financial issues yourself, due to loss of a job, divorce or just plain overspending, you may want to rethink the joint account issue so that you're not tempted to dip into the pot for your own benefit. And if your parent is still able to manage for themselves, a joint account is really not necessary. But it is something to think about. Check with the bank.

And you may want to have $15,000 in savings or checking (**liquid assets**) for immediate use. While that may seem exorbitant, believe me, when your parent requires medications, has doctor's bills, nursing home costs and medical equipment needs, you'll want immediate access to anywhere from $5000 to $10,000. For example: while **Medicare** often will reimburse you, in part or in whole, for doctor recommended equipment, you may have to pay out-of-pocket if you want immediate delivery. And an assisted living facility or nursing home will often want one month's rent in advance and that could amount to over $5000.

Again, you can see why it's a good thing to encourage your parent to assign the same person who is **POA** to be **executor** of the will. The POA should be familiar with the needs, bills, personal contacts, and their parent's financial situation. *(Be sure to fill out the forms in chapter 14)*

You will, of course, be held accountable for any money used from your parent's account—so keep receipts. Label the receipts with the name of the article you purchased and make notations in their checkbook register and the memo on the check itself that explains what the purchase was for.

Doctors and hospitals can take months to get their bills out to you and so you need to keep the deceased parent's bank account open at least six months to a year, until all matters are settled. After that, if there are other heirs, the remainder of the joint account should be distributed according to the will.

CHAPTER 4

MEDICAL:
Doctor, Hospital, Nursing Home, Hospice

(Discuss the following information with the medical professionals)

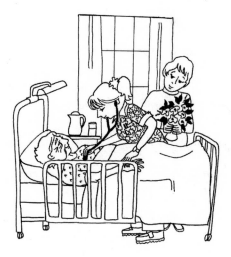

Your parent's good health is essential to how well they can fulfill their senior dreams. Their good health reduces the expensive medical bills which might otherwise destroy their joy, savings and your eventual inheritance. So finding good care and keeping them well is a win-win all the way around.

Whether your Mom and Dad want to enjoy time with their grandchildren and family or be active in community programs, want to take that long-awaited trip around the country in a camper or go cruising through the Caribbean, your parent will need good health care. And since outpatient surgery, medications and dental work can put a crimp in anyone's budget, especially a senior on a fixed income, it is imperative that you make certain your parent has adequate insurance coverage.

In chapters 5 and 6, I will go into more detail about the benefits of **Medicare, Medicaid** and **insurances** in general, but for now, I will encourage you to go over any medical coverage that your parent's former employer may have allowed them to keep. **Be sure all policies are paid up to date and are still in effect after your parent turns 65.** And carefully go over what their primary insurance (*normally Medicare Part A and B, Medicare Part C, or a Medicare supplement*) covers (*hospital, out-patient, medications, doctor office visits, lab testing, dental, hearing aids, eye care, etc.*)

That said, let's look at the areas of concern to your parent in the medical field.

Doctor or Nurse Practitioner

It's a good idea to talk to your parent's doctor or **nurse practitioner,** even if you have to schedule an office appointment. With legal **POA papers for the health care** of your parent, you will be able to change doctors, question medications or surgical procedures and change nursing homes—if you feel it's necessary.

Be careful that you don't abuse your powers and, more importantly, be sure you are upholding the wishes of your parent. And keep your siblings informed of any decisions to alter your parent's care to ensure you keep that "all-important" *peace* in the family.

IMPORTANT

Get **DNR*** (Do Not Resuscitate) papers drawn up by the doctor or nurse practitioner. There are 2 kinds of DNR to choose from, DNR-cc and DNR-arrest.

*check the definitions for **"DNR-cc"** or **"DNR-arrest"** in chapter 8

Do be sure that your parent has a doctor who is familiar with geriatric care and makes your parent feel comfortable. Also, don't be surprised if your parent will require more than one doctor. They will need a regular family practitioner, an optometrist (for their eye care), they may require hearing aides and even a chiropractor (for their back or joint problems).

Having a good rapport with your parent's doctors may mean better treatment and peace of mind for everyone. When a concerned family member, especially one who has POA credentials, visits regularly and inquires about their parent, statistics have shown that the patient often receives more attention by the staff. And when a family member gives compliments and thank-you gifts to the medical staff in a hospital or nursing home, it often reaps the benefit of better care for the patient.

In order for you to know exactly what your parent's wishes are—converse often. Talk after a new health problem or health issues which may have arisen in their aging friend's life. Sometimes, as health problems increase, your parent may change their staunchly held opinion against surgery or alternative medicines. Because your parent may be weakened from an illness or feel less empowered in their old age, you may need to speak for them. *(For a list of helpful topics to discuss with your parent, check out chapter 14.)*

Talk to the doctor and ask questions until you fully understand the consequences of the treatment being prescribed. Sometimes doctor's explanations may be a bit difficult to understand, so ask questions and try to interpret what the doctor is saying to your parent so they will understand and trust the doctor.

Be brief and honest, while still giving your parent the most positive slant on the procedure, so your parent will feel hopeful as they face surgery or chemotherapy. Hope, after all, is an important part of their healing process. And hope is even important in the dying process, which I'll discuss in *chapter 12.*

To be sure that your parent is getting the best treatment, record all their medical information; allergies, medications they are presently taking, their health history and the health history of their family, etc. *(I have provided health forms for you to fill out in chapter 14, and a convenient wallet-sized version of the information in chapter 11.)*

If your parent is in a nursing home, you may be dealing more with a nurse practitioner than you will with the actual doctor in charge of your parent's case.

A nurse practitioner is what it sounds like, a registered nurse with additional training as a doctor. With doctors checking on hospital patients in the morning, office patients in the afternoon, and checking on a multitude of elderly patients in the nursing home towards evening—the nurse practitioner serves as a liaison between the patient and the doctor. And you can get DNR (Do Not Resuscitate papers) as well as any medication prescription authorizations drawn up by a doctor or nurse practitioner.

IMPORTANT

Request a **Handicap Tag** from the doctor for your car. It will allow you to park closer to the curb when transporting your parent.

WARNING: Don't leave the tag on your visor while driving, for visibility reasons, and use it only when required.

Though **DNR** papers seem to be foreboding, they can save a lot of grief. They mean what they say. You're asking the doctor and EMS personnel to not use any CPR tactics like; chest compressions, electric paddles or heart massage. It can be very traumatic to vigorously push on an 85-year-old patient's chest when their bones are brittle and their skin is thin and fragile. And getting zapped with an electrically charged paddle is no picnic either.

While **Do Not Resuscitate** may sound indifferent and cold, you're actually doing your parent a favor. If a heart attack patient is in his forties or fifties, he should be able to endure the treatment and recover in a reasonable length of time, but when that patient is in their 80's or 90's, they could suffer a punctured lung, a fractured rib or they could be badly bruised and bed-ridden for weeks or months from the trauma. Think about it. Talk it over with your parent and doctor.

How do you shop for the right doctor? Ask other patients and friends in your church or community. Sometimes a nurse or nursing home personnel will offer his/her opinion.

Hospitals

So many treatments and surgeries are done in the doctor's office or as outpatients today that it is very rare to actually need a lengthy hospital stay. And even then, patients are usually released from the hospital in a matter of days. So it is important that your parent's insurance policy covers outpatient surgery as well as hospital stays and rehabilitation time in a nursing home.

TRUE STORY

My father was treated for heart failure in a large hospital in Pittsburgh. Unfortunately, the only help they could give him was Lasix and oxygen. After he moved to a small town adjacent to a retirement community, the doctor recommended prostate surgery. After the surgery, he was able to have three more active years of life.

MORAL: Don't be afraid of a small hospital and don't be afraid to change doctors.

Because of the advancements in laser surgery, many operations that were once considered serious are becoming less threatening and the recovery time is greatly reduced as well. Ask around for the best hospital and doctor for any procedure your parent may need and don't be starry-eyed by the size of the hospital or the credentials on the doctor's wall. Often a small hospital near a retirement community is more aware and capable of treating seniors than large metropolitan hospitals.

If you are new to the area, ask advice of the long-time residents in that area that have had to go to the hospital in question. Inquire at work or in your place of worship. Often older members have had surgeries and visited friends who have gone to various hospitals. Be sure your parent's insurance will cover procedures for that hospital and doctor. In some cases, they will only accept their insurance coverage in an emergency. *(Check chapters 5, 6, and 8.)*

Nursing Homes

Aging parents dread them and their children feel guilty about sending their parents to them, but nursing homes have given undeniable comfort and help to the patient that needs them. While we will be talking about the nursing home issue again in *chapters 9 and 10*, let's go over some of the issues right now.

What Nursing Homes are NOT . . .

- They are **not** foster homes for the aged, a place to dump your parents when you don't want them around anymore.

- They are **not** a poorly-staffed poorly-cared for place for unloved souls.
- They are **not** a place to die.
- They are **not** a place to be avoided by the family.

What Nursing Homes are . . .

- They **are** staffed by round-the-clock skilled registered nurses and other caring staff, trained in the area of geriatrics.
- They **are** a safe place for your dementia or handicapped parent to live.
- They **are** a place where trained activities directors plan daily crafts, musical interaction and even outdoor trips.
- They **are** a temporary place for rehabilitation from strokes and other physical problems.
- They **are** a place for you and your family to visit frequently and create a personal outreach to other patients who may have fewer visitors.

How to find a good nursing home . . .

- Check the internet for the facility's rating. **www.carescout.com**
- Ask friends with a parent in a nursing home, hospital personnel or nursing home staff for their opinion of their establishment.
- Visit several times, unexpectedly. Don't be discouraged if there is an occasional odor. After all, there are probably 20 or more adults in diapers. Notice the attentiveness of the nurses and aides. Do they smile? Do they speak in loving terms, like "sweetie" and "honey" or even give a gentle hug when they walk by them in the hall?
- Talk to your church's outreach group or individuals that visit the nursing homes. Get their opinion of the one you plan to set up your parent in and even join the outreach group to get familiar with local nursing homes.
- Check if the facility accepts Medicaid patients, just in case your parent may require a long stay or they've run out of funds. Do realize that there are conditions to receiving Medicaid. Check **www.medicaid.com** site and chapter 5.
- Look around. Prices and accommodations vary greatly. You can expect to pay $5000 a month for just a room and meals. On top of the room will be medications, doctor visits and any tests or hospital visits and it may not include laundry. It may sound like a lot of money, but if your

parent has long-term care insurance, Social Security, a house to sell and investments, you should be able to handle it. (While most patients only live about 3 years or less in a nursing home, Alzheimer's patients can be there for 6 years or more. President Reagan was in a nursing home for ten years. So be cautious with your parent's finances.)

Hospice

If you're like me, I only heard a couple of stories about hospice before requiring their services. In fact, I never really knew what they did, except that they helped people who were dying. Well, there's a lot more to it than that.

Hospice is the name of the nationwide organization that assists in "end-of-life" issues, but each state and city will have a group of hospice workers who identify themselves by their own unique names and care options, like Incare, Harbor Light, Heartland Home Care or Mount Carmel Hospice out of Columbus, Ohio.

To find a hospice group for your parent . . .

- Look up **Hospice** in the Yellow Pages.
- Ask for a recommendation from the hospital or nursing home.
- To find the hospice nearest you, go to . . . **www.hospicenet.org**

If you find your parent in a very serious health situation, but not necessarily dying, give hospice a call. They'll decide if your parent is eligible.

And don't worry about the cost. Hospice is fully covered by **Medicare** and many hospices have been known to absorb the costs of non-Medicare patients. You have nothing to lose and everything to gain by just one phone call.

What will most HOSPICES do for you and your parent?

- Give comfort care for your parent, if they have a life-limiting illness.
- Help to control symptoms and offer pain management.
- Reduce your out-of-pocket expenses by supplying pain medications, medical equipment and services for FREE.
- Offer care to the burdened and often grieving family.
- Offer spiritual, emotional, and financial counseling support to you and your parent.

- Give you the peace of mind that hospice nurses and counselors are available to make visits or answer calls 24 hours a day, even if your parent is already in a nursing home facility.
- Continued counseling help for the family going through the bereavement process, even after the death of your parent.
- Personal care. (bathing, feeding, dressing)
- Care given out of your parent's home, a nursing home or a hospice care facility.
- Dietary help.
- Physician care.
- Physical therapy, speech therapy and occupational therapy.

TRUE STORY

My 90-year-old mother was in a nursing home when they discovered she had developed bleeding ulcers in her stomach and esophagus. The trauma of the invasive procedure was too much for her and I inquired about hospice. Although my mother recovered from her ulcer, hospice remained vigilant at the nursing home and was there for us when she had two bad falls that left her with a broken arm and hip. Hospice comforted the entire family, provided medications and equipment to make my mother comfortable right up to her death, nine months after we had initially called them. Their presence really helped me through the awkward moments at the end of my mother's life.

MORAL: Don't hesitate to call hospice, even if you don't think the problem is serious enough. You'll be glad you did!

CHAPTER 5

Medicare and Medicaid

(Discuss the following information with the insurance professionals.)

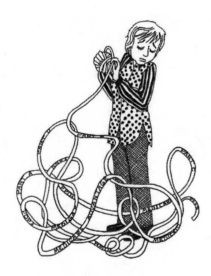

There are so many Medicare Advantage and Medigap plans out there that you may feel overwhelmed. That's how I felt as I approached my 65th birthday. Then I decided to find some answers and so I began to read.

I read the actual advertisements for the various Medicare plans; I even interviewed a broker for Medicare insurance and read over the Medicare and Medicaid websites. Based on all my research, I can only tell you that each person's needs determine which plan is best for him or her. Here are my findings, as of 2011, in regards to **Medicare, Medigap, Medicare prescription drug plans** and **Medicare Advantage** plans as well as **Medicaid**.

Medicare

If your parent has received their Medicare Card, you may be wondering why they need to be concerned about their medical coverage.

Doesn't Medicare take care of the elderly? And if so, why are there so many Medicare supplements out there?

All eligible seniors receive a Medicare card when they reach age 65.

What does Medicare cover?

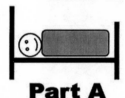

Part A

Inpatient hospital stay ● short stay in nursing home ● hospice ● some home health care

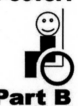

Part B

Outpatient surgery ● doctor visits ● lab testing● preventative services

So why do you need Part C, Part D, or Medigap?

 Part C

In place of your Medicare Part A and B is **Part C** (also known as a **Medicare Advantage Plan**) which provides everything Part A and B does.

DISADVANTAGES:
● You have to go to the doctor or hospital in that Part C plan. Either ____ PPO or PFFS.
● You may have an extra monthly fee

ADVANTAGES:
● You often get extra bonuses, like prescription drug discounts, Silver Sneakers health program, eye care, etc..

 Part D

Part D, PDPs, or **Prescription Drug Plans** are available to help pay for all the medications your parent may need.

DISADVANTAGES:
● You will incur a monthly fee.

ADVANTAGES:
● You can reduce your monthly medication costs.

**Do check if their medications are already greatly reduced by Kroger, Walmart, etc. pharmacy. Many generic drugs can be purchased for only $4 a month.

MEDIGAP

Medigap or **Medicare Supplemental Insurance** is what it sounds like. It fills the "gap" between what Medicare Part A, B or C covers and what your parent may need.

DISADVANTAGES:
● You will incur a monthly fee, usually larger than Part C.

ADVANTAGES:
● You will be receiving a reduction in dental, optical, and/ or hearing aid costs.

*Never get rid of your original Medicare Card, even if you sign up for other plans.

First of all, let's get some definitions straight. It's essential to your decision as to which plan is best for your parent. Since your 65year-old (or older) parent will receive primary medical coverage through Medicare or a Medicare Advantage Plan, let's take a look at what those are. Check the websites of each provider to see what new coverages may be available: **medicare.com, medicare. gov, medicare.org, medicaid.com** and **medicaid.org**

What are Medicare Part A, B, C, D, and Medigap?

- **Medicare:** This is a government-funded medical care program for eligible seniors, who are 65 or older. Anyone who is months away from their 65th birthday will receive their Medicare card and information in the mail. (Hang onto the card, even if you pick another plan.)

- **Medicare Part A:** This **inpatient hospital coverage** is automatically a part of your parent's Medicare package. Part A is what your parent is entitled to when they get their Medicare card. **It's FREE.** (Well, truth is your folks have been paying for it out of their paycheck for years). Part A helps cover their inpatient stay in the hospital, short stays in a skilled nursing home facility, hospice care and some home health care. It doesn't cover everything but it does pay for a goodly portion of it.

If you want additional coverage for the hospital bills that Medicare doesn't pay, you'll want to look into **Medigap** Insurance. And if you want coverage for outpatient surgery and lab tests, then you'll want to consider **Medicare Part B**, because Part A doesn't cover that stuff. Part A also doesn't cover medications, dental work, hearing aids or eyeglasses. For more coverage, you'll want to look into **Part C** and **D**. Are you completely bumfuzzled yet? Take a little time to go over my Medicare chart on the previous page.

- **Medicare Part B:** This **outpatient medical coverage** needs to be elected by your parent as an addition to their Medicare Part A plan. It will cost your parent **an extra sum of money each month** but they will be adding the following services to their coverage: outpatient medical and surgical services (very common surgical procedures today), laboratory testing, limited home health care and preventative services such as flu shots, bone mass testing, hepatitis B shots, mammograms, etc. Good idea to get this plan right from the start.

IMPORTANT

You MUST sign up for Medicare Part A and Part B in a timely fashion BEFORE you can elect Part C, D or Medigap.

- **Medicare Part C:** Part C is a combination of Medicare Part A (inpatient hospital coverage), Medicare Part B (outpatient medical coverage) and Part D (Prescription Drug Plan) combined. It's also called **Medicare Advantage**. With Part C, you will no longer need the typical Medicare Part A and Part B . . . but DON'T throw away your Medicare card. Tuck it away in a safe place for future use. Yes, most Medicare Part C programs **will cost your parent a small monthly fee** but that's because they cover more than Medicare Part A and Part B.

How does Part C do more for just a little extra money each month? They find PPOs and PFFS plans that can get the same medical care for less than standard Medicare.

The Part C plans are purchased through a Medicare-approved insurance company. Unlike a normal Medicare plan, your parent must see doctors that are within the plan (**PPOs, PFFS**)* The advantages are that your parent may spend less out-of-pocket. * *Don't worry if you don't know what these terms mean, all the bold printed terms will be defined later in this chapter and again in chapter 8.*

- **Medicare Part D:** This is a Medicare prescription drug plan, also known as a **PDP** (**P**rescription **D**rug **P**lan) and **MAPD** (**M**edicare **A**dvantage **P**rescription **D**rug **P**lan), that is available to everyone with Medicare, but it is purchased through a private company or insurance company that is Medicare-approved. Your parent chooses the Medicare drug plan that seems right for them and **they will have to pay a monthly premium**. Your parent can join a Medicare drug plan 3 months after they begin their Medicare coverage. Also, your parent can change their Medicare drug plan later on.

- **Medigap:** This is a Medicare Supplemental Insurance policy that will help pay for the stuff that Medicare doesn't cover—but they **must be enrolled in Medicare Part A and Part B** in order to qualify for Medigap. You'll still need to consider a prescription drug plan though. And, yep, **your parent will be paying extra** for Medigap. Which doctor you choose depends on whether or not the doctor accepts Medicare—which most do.

Summation of Medicare and Medigap

Everyone who is eligible for Medicare and who turned 65 will receive a Medicare Card in the mail, which will cover a portion of their hospital expenses and nursing home care. That's **Part A** coverage. It's a FREE coverage that your parent will automatically receive.

If your parent decides to increase that coverage to **Part B**, which is highly recommended, they may do so through Medicare at the time they receive their card. This will give them partial coverage for out-patient surgeries and preventative services, like flu shots. All doctors and hospitals accept Part A and Part B, but Part B is not free. It requires an additional monthly fee.

Part C, also known as a **Medicare Advantage Plan**, is just another way of saying your parent can change the Medicare Part A and B coverage AFTER they've signed up for them and then opt to pick up their own Medicare-approved health care insurance plan that will cover everything Part A and B does, plus a little more, and it costs a little less. The catch is that not all doctors or hospitals will accept the conditions of Part C coverages—unless it's an emergency. These plans usually are attached to **PPOs, PFFS,** or **SNPs**. *(We'll get to just what those initials stand for in a minute.)*

So go over these Part C plans through **medicare.com** and **medicare.gov**. This website will list and compare the plans via an easy-to-understand chart. Since your parent may not be computer savvy, you may want to print out the charts, circle the ones you think best suit them and then sit down with your parent to discuss each plan's advantages and disadvantages.

IMPORTANT

Hang onto your parent's original Medicare Card, no matter what other plan they may opt for.

Part D is just for prescription drug discounts. Sometimes a Part C plan will include a prescription drug plan, so they don't need Part D. But if your parent opts for Medicare Part A and Part B, they really should consider Part D, too.

Once again, check out **www.Medicare.com** for a listing of all the prescription drug plans. The good news is that your parent can shift this plan around to suit their changing health needs.

IMPORTANT

Do not keep switching plans, or you may find your parent is without coverage due to start up dates or previous conditions, just when they need it the most.

And if you feel content that you and your parent have made the right decision, about which way to go with Medicare Part A, Part B, Part C, and Part D—consider an addition to the whole can of worms they call **Medigap Insurance**.

Medigap insurance is what your parent may need to pay the extra cost of any hospital stay. Part A pays for some of the inpatient hospital costs and Part B pays for some of the out-patient costs, but Medigap picks up most of what those policies *don't* cover. Your parent will have 6 months, after they turn 65 and get enrolled in Part B, to sign up for Medigap insurance. After that time frame, if they should then decide they want Medigap, they may have to pay more for the policy.

There are several Medigap insurance policies to choose from, labeled A, B, C, D . . . well, you get the picture. And each policy will offer a different coverage. A covers more than B and B covers more than C. Of course, the more the coverage, the more your parent will have to pay for the insurance. Talk to your parent's insurance agent or insurance broker to check out their Medigap options.

I know that your parent's income is probably fixed and greatly reduced from their earlier earning years. Plus they are now faced with additional expenses for medical coverage. And if your parent is in good health, they may feel this whole health coverage worry is just a scam to get their money. It is frustrating.

However, since most of us tend to need more medical attention as we grow older, I know I do, consider the various policies carefully. With rising health costs and reduced income, medical bills can quickly reduce your parent's estate.

On the other hand, unnecessary insurances could reduce their present standard of living. It's a lot to think about. But don't despair, any decision you make is better than none and most of them can be reversed.

By the way, if your parent has special needs, there are 3 Medicare Special Needs options to choose from. Check out the **www.Medicare.com** listing for more details.

Even though we are talking about Medicare stuff here, I do want you to consider another health coverage policy that may be vital to your parent's future care. **Long-Term Care Insurance** could really help if your parent is ever in need of skilled nursing level care in assisted living, nursing home or in-home care. With seniors living longer and especially if Alzheimer's runs in your family, Long-Term Care insurance could be a real blessing.

Hopefully your parent was able to secure the **dental coverage plan** from their previous place of employment.

Well here we go again, back to a list of definitions. Only these have to do with the doctor and hospital coverage for **Medicare Advantage Plans**, or what we have also referred to as **Part C**.

What are these PPO, PFSS and SNP plans?

- **PPOs** With the **P**referred **P**rovider **O**rganization plan, **PPO** for short, you can go to specialists without referrals, but you pay more if you go to doctors or hospitals outside the plan's network, except in emergencies.
- **PFFS plans** This plan**, P**rivate **F**ee-**F**or-**S**ervice plan, allows you to go to any doctor or hospital that will accept the terms of that plan. A doctor or hospital can accept the plan one time and reject it another time, except in an emergency.
- **SNPs** This **S**pecial **N**eeds **P**lan, is only for people in long-term care facilities who receive both Medicaid and Medicare or have certain illnesses or disabilities.

Since Social Security and Medicare are such hot topics in our political arena today, it's likely that we will see these facts change over the next five years. Let's hope they become less confusing and less expensive, but I'm not going to hold my breath. Meanwhile, keep asking questions of your insurance agent.

What about MEDICAID?

- **Medicaid:** While Medicaid sounds a lot like Medicare, it is really quite different. Medicaid is also a government run program and it will cover the costs for inpatient and outpatient hospital care, nursing home care and medications, but ALL seniors are NOT illegible for Medicaid. Medicaid is limited to persons who are in the low income level or have special needs that require a lot of extra medical attention. Check out **www.Medicaid.com** for more up-to-date information.

CHAPTER 6

INSURANCE:
Life, Home, Car, Long Term Care

(Discuss the following information with the insurance professionals)

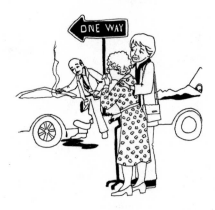

Insurance Agent

There are several things you need to go over with your parent's insurance agent and it's also a good idea to share the agent's game plan with your parent's financial planner. It's kind of like the government's checks and balances. Congress checks on the President, the Senate checks on the House of Representatives, and the Supreme Court checks on all of them. So think of the financial planner as a check on the insurance agent . . . and vice versa . . . and you and your parent as the final say in the matter.

Questions . . .

- **Do my parents have, or need, life insurance?**

  While that may seem like an unusual question to ask, a single senior parent who has a very large nest egg with no mortgage, at-home children *or outstanding bills probably doesn't need to be spending more money on additional life insurance policies. If your parent still has debts to pay, a small **term life** insurance policy may help reduce that debt until it is paid off or they may want to leave a "tax-free" inheritance for their heirs via a **whole life** insurance policy. (Talk to their insurance agent.)*

- **What kind of** life insurance **do they have—or need? (Whole Life or Term Life?)**

*Remember, **whole life** will be there for them until they die and if they want to borrow on it, there is some money in there for them to take out. It costs more than **term life**. However, if they only have a critical window of time that they are worried about paying off a mortgage or they still have children at home, they may want to buy into **term life** because it's cheaper. The down side is that term life cuts off after a given age that's stated in the policy. At that point, the policy is closed and yields nothing. Also, you can't draw money out of a term life policy and term life may be too costly for a senior, due to their age. (Talk to their insurance agent about these points.)*

- **Are your parents over-insured?**

Your parent may have old policies that they've forgotten about or been pressured into buying. Policies they don't need. If your parent is still paying premiums, check the conditions of the policies to be sure they are appropriate for your parent's situation.

- **Should they cash out a policy?**

If they want to cash in a life insurance policy to go on a cruise or like my one grandmother, who cashed her life insurance policy in for gambling money . . . try to stop them. However, if they fit into the category of the "over insured," do look into reducing their policies and thus their premiums. (More stuff to ask the agent about.)

- **Do they have a Medicare supplemental insurance?**

There are lots of plans to choose from, so get informed. Also, know that your parent can change their supplemental after a year if they decide it isn't working well for them. (More Medicare information in Chapter 5.)

- **Do they have a Long Term Care policy?**

Long Term Care insurance is available to anyone 80-years-old or younger, who is in decent health. The older you are when you get it, the more it costs, but it could be a blessing to someone who may need assisted living or nursing home care in the future. Be sure the policy includes an in-home nursing care option and comes from a reputable company. Check around, policies vary in price and coverage.

Remember, hospice is available to all Medicare recipients for free—in a nursing home, a hospice facility or their own home—but the health issues need to be life-threatening, not Alzheimer's or wheelchair-bound patients.

- **Do they have adequate car insurance? And if they have given up their car, have you dropped their car insurance?**

The cost of elevated insurance for an elderly driver who has had frequent tickets, minor or major accidents can be one of the signs that tell you it may be time to give up the car. Remind your parent that this is not just an issue of their independence but also the lives of other drivers and pedestrians.

If your parent is still driving well, be sure they have adequate insurance and consider adding an **umbrella policy***.*

- **Do they have home or apartment insurance? Be sure to explain where your parent lives.** (Retirement housing, assisted living, nursing home resident.)

Nursing homes and assisted living facilities may have some coverage for lost or damaged items or you may want to insure valuable items, such as a flat-screen TV, but generally speaking, these housing areas are too sparsely furnished to require insurance.

- **Would it be wise to get my parent an umbrella insurance to protect them against law suits?**

This "personal umbrella" insurance is a good idea for anyone who is living in their own home and/or owns a car. It will protect against any major law suits if your parent gets in a car accident or someone falls on their icy steps. There is even a "commercial umbrella" insurance for their business, if they have one. (It will **not** cover slander or defamation of character law suites.)

- Ask about a final expense policy or funeral insurance to pay for funeral expenses, if they have not done a prepaid funeral plan with the funeral home. It can't be touched by Medicaid if your parent becomes financially indigent.

TRUE STORY

When my parents moved into their retirement community, my mother was 80. She had high blood pressure and some problems with arthritis but it didn't stop her from getting a **long term care plan**. My father had decided on a three-year coverage for her, which meant she would receive a monthly income for only three years in a special care facility. I didn't begin to use the coverage until she was 88, in assisted living. One year later, she was assigned to a nursing home, where we used up the final 2-year coverage. Six months later, she died. Between Social Security, a meager pension, and Long Term Care coverage, my mother only needed an extra $1500 a month to pay for her $5500 room, medications, and doctor bills. I made an automatic withdrawal from her investments to cover that expense. $1500 was a lot better than an extra $3900.

MORAL: Long Term Care policies are getting harder to obtain, but if you can find one with a reputable company and a reasonable fee and your parent is eligible, they can be a good investment. (Talk to their insurance agent and see how other coverages have faired over the last ten years for other long term care policy holders. Have premiums kept going up or coverage kept going down . . . or has it stayed pretty much the same?)

CHAPTER 7

FUNERALS:
Preplanned/Prepaid

(Discuss the following information with the funeral director)

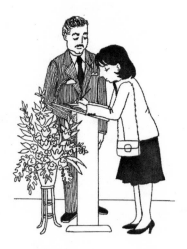

There I go again, with still another unpleasant subject—funerals. But it can be even more unpleasant if it is left to the normal three-day window of preparation that is allotted to the bereaved, after the death of their loved one.

If you don't prepare ahead of time, in just thirty-six hours or less you will need to select the following:

(1)   Funeral home.
(2)   Casket.
(3)   Burial site.
(4)   Headstone.
(5)   Clothes to be worn by the deceased at the viewing.
(6)   Music which may include special musicians or vocalists.
(7)   Locating a particular group or organization that your parent had supported and preferred donations to over flowers.

(8) List of names of friends or loved ones that need to be notified.

(9) Picture for the announcement in the newspaper and the funeral home director.

(10) Obituary for the newspaper (Many papers charge for obituaries).

(11) Program for the funeral home to distribute during the viewing and funeral.

(12) Special internment requests, such as a twenty-one gun salute for a military veteran.

(13) Clergyman to speak at the funeral service and internment (it's customary to give a donation for his/her service).

Need I say more? Look over my checklist for funerals in *chapter 14* and start answering all the questions well in advance.

Hopefully, you'll be able to openly talk to your parent about what they would like to have done for their funeral. The funeral home refers to it as a **preplanned funeral**, which can also be **prepaid**.

In a **prepaid funeral** with the funeral home, the funeral director can arrange for all the details to your parent's specifications, so you don't have to rehash it in the midst of your grieving. If your parent has elected to have a prepaid funeral, the funeral home should put their money in a **trust** that will lock your parent's funeral expenses into today's rates. Your parent may also opt for a **final expense policy** with your parent's insurance agent. (*Talk over the advantages of either option with the funeral home director and the insurance agent.*)

TRUE STORY

My mother sat down with the funeral director and planned out nearly every phase of her funeral, soon after my father's death, even though she was perfectly healthy. Mom surprised me as she enthusiastically selected her casket as if she were at a furniture store picking out a sofa. She even chose the casket bouquet that she preferred. I'm grateful for my mother's ability to plan out all the particulars of her funeral, eight years ahead of the fact, because it made our period of mourning less distracted by time-consuming details.

MORAL: Don't be frightened about the thought of preplanning your parent's funeral and do encourage them to do that, even if they don't prepay.

My mother not only preplanned her funeral but she also paid for it in advance. While **preplanned funerals** (laying out all the details that your parent wants for their funeral) is an excellent thing to do, **prepaid funerals** should be well researched. Interview the funeral director and insurance agent and then review their answers with your parent's financial advisor before finalizing your decision.

Things to question the funeral director, insurance agent and financial consultant about . . .

- How well established is the funeral home that your parent is considering?
- How much does the funeral home charge for their services?
- What factors can affect the final bill of the funeral? (Flowers, long distance transportation of the body, etc.)
- How is the funeral home investing the money for a prepaid funeral*? (Ask your insurance agent about a **final expense policy** or **funeral insurance***)
- If your parent elects cremation and a private distribution of the ashes, is a prepaid plan even necessary?
- Is your parent young enough and invested well enough to make more from their investments than from the funeral homes investment of their prepaid funeral funds?
- Why should your parent prepay to the funeral home instead of purchasing a **funeral insurance*** from their insurance company?
- What would happen if you had to move your parent to another town . . . would the original agreement still hold?

* *Remember, prepaid funerals and funeral insurance policies are not taxable and cannot be touched by Medicaid if your parent should require their services.*

Plan to provide an enjoyable life now, for your parent, and an honorable recognition of them after they pass away. You probably have children, maybe grandchildren, a job, and perhaps other invalids to care for but work your parents into your weekly or monthly plans. As they become a part of your routine, you will feel less burdened. *(Be sure to go over all the questions about funerals in chapter 14, with your parent and the funeral director.)*

IMPORTANT

Since you'll need a lot of **original death certificates** to close accounts with Social Security, pension benefits, any investments, insurance companies, banks, etc., ask the funeral home to order about **eight** or **ten** death certificates.

Each certificate can cost between $2 to $20 or more, depending on what state your parent lived in at the time of their death. But getting the death certificates right after the funeral is a lot easier than going to the county court house, where your parent died during rush hour or having to wait for the mail to deliver them. Been there . . . done that.

CHAPTER 8
DICTIONARY:
Cutting Through the Mumbo Jumbo

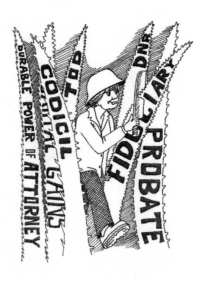

DEFINITIONS of TERMS and PERSONS pertaining to:
● FINANCIAL ● LEGAL and **● HEALTH** matters

The first seven definitions are to help you understand who the persons are that you need to talk to and the remainder of the dictionary defines terms relevant to three important caregivng topics: (1) financial and insurance (2) medical and (3) legal. Some terms may be repeated under each of the topics in order to help you locate the definitions quickly when you are meeting with the professional in that field.

Accountant or CPA: This person has studied tax laws and can quickly understand your parent's tax issues. He can even help your parent decide when to best **gift** money and how many legitimate **deductions** your parent can declare. This person will charge for the services he has rendered, while most simple questions that can be answered over the phone will not incur a charge. Ask about their charges before using their services. *(More about this person in chapter 3)*

Doctor: MD, OS, holistic, nurse practitioner, optometrist, dentist, or whatever title of the physician, your parent will need a doctor—probably more than one. And getting a doctor who works well with the geriatric set can be tricky, so you may want to ask for a recommendation from a neighboring nursing home. Be sure the doctor accepts your parent's medical coverage plan: **HMOs, PPOs, PFFs,** and **SNPs.** While most doctors will talk to the designated POA over the phone, for free, some may require that you come in during your parent's office appointment or schedule an appointment just for consultation. *(More about doctors in chapter 4)*

Estate lawyer or Eldercare lawyer: An estate lawyer understands **Elder Law.** He covers things like: **wills, living wills, trusts** and concerns for the **estate** of your parent and his/her **heirs.** He can draw up the necessary paperwork and offer some advice. Remember, attorneys do not come cheap. Many will even charge for a phone consultation as short as five minutes. So ask about their fees before you make an appointment. *(More about this person in chapters 2 and 15)*

Financial planner, consultant or advisor: This is a professional person who looks out for your parent's investments. This person can set up an **investment portfolio** for your parent, give advice as to the *need* of a **will, living will** or **trust,** check if your parent has a **long term care** plan, adequate **liquid assets** and more. While they can sign your parent up for **mutual funds, annuities,** etc., they do *not* draw up official elder care papers, like wills and trusts. Once your parent is a client and you are established as their POA, you should be able to meet with your parent's financial planner as often as you have questions, for free. *(More about this person in chapters 3 and 15)*

Funeral director: Also called a mortician or undertaker, this is the person in charge of the funeral home and all the funeral arrangements. Your parent may want to set up a **preplanned** or **prepaid funeral.** Since funerals can cost over $7000, many seniors like to pay for them ahead of time to lock into today's prices and know they will have the funeral of their choosing. Check the reputation and longevity of the funeral home before investing and run the proposed expenses by your parent's financial advisor. Also consider talking to their insurance agent about a **funeral insurance policy.**

Hospice personnel: This caring support group of dedicated nurses, counselors and pastors are available, free of charge to Medicare patients, to assist you in the time of your parent's most crucial health issues. They will come to your parent's home, a care facility or even bring your parent into their hospice facility. Hospice provides comfort, encouragement, nursing care, medications, information to the patient and the caregiver and even spiritual guidance. Each hospice unit has a different name, so you may want to ask the hospital, local nursing home or check under Hospice in the yellow pages to connect you to one in your area. Don't overlook the value of this service in your care giving duties. And remember, you don't have to wait until your parent is on their deathbed. Hospice is there to serve during any critical health issues. *(Check out chapter 4 and 15)*

Insurance agent: This professional has studied all the advantages and disadvantages of **insurances** and **annuities** and can even help in the area of **financial planning.** They will let you know if you are over insured or if a **term life** policy may be better than a **whole life.** They can even set your parent up with a **long-term care plan, Medicare Advantage** or **Medigap policy** and **funeral insurance.** *(More about this person and Medicare in Chapters 5 and 6)*

❶   Financial & Insurance Terms

401K or 403B or 457 : Check **SEP**

Annuities: Under an annuity contract with an insurance company, you make an up-front payment or series of payments, and anticipate a stream of income in their retirement years. So, in essence, an annuity is a savings account with your insurance agency or investment company. Your earnings are tax-deferred until you remove the money. Annuities come in several forms; **fixed** and **variable.**

Assets: Assets are anything that has a tangible value. Your parent's house, car, boat, stocks, bonds, cash, quality jewelry, antiques, collectables, savings account, checking account, business and life insurance policy are all assets. Most furniture, clothing, and memorabilia are not considered assets.

If your parent had taken out several loans or used a lot of credit cards, their debt may be bigger than their assets. Try to calculate their total assets and then their total debt. Which is more? That's their true value.

Bear Market: You will hear bear and bull market from your financial planner a lot. A bear market simply refers to a slow financial market often noted by a severe drop in the **DOW** numbers, which usually indicates that your investments are going down.

Beneficiaries or heirs: That's the name given to someone who benefits, in money or things, from the death of someone else. In other words, if you're named as a beneficiary in your parent's life insurance policy, investments, will or trust, then you're one of the heirs due to receive the assets. There may be more than one beneficiary or heir, especially if your parent has more than one child. Beneficiaries can also be grandchildren, a church, a nonprofit organization, a friend or even a pet.

Bonds: These are certificates that you can purchase from the government or a corporation that guarantees the original cost of the document, plus the interest they promised by a specified date. They are usually secure; at least they are as secure as the group you purchased them from.

If you buy a **bond fund**, through your mutual funds, you will find that they will fluctuate. There is no guarantee of their value. They are a good purchase when stocks are down however their value can go down when stocks are up. Check with your financial planner.

Bull Market: Like the above bear market, you will hear this term in the financial sector of your work as a **POA**. If you do hear that we are in a bull market, that's good. It means the **DOW** readings are usually going up and we have a good economic outlook. It also means your parent's investments are probably going up, too.

Capital Gains: When an investment is cashed in after the death of your parent, the amount of money it made, from the day your parent died to the time that you cashed it, is called "capital gains".

*EXAMPLE: Let's say your parent had IBM stocks worth $10,000, at the time of their death. If you cashed in the stocks at $10,000, you would NOT owe capital gain taxes. However, if you waited for 6 months, after your parent passed away, and the stock rose to $12,000 in value, you would owe taxes on the added $2,000 value (which is the capital gain). Of course, if the stock did not gain in value over the 6 month period after your parent's death, or even lost money, you would **not** have had any capital gain.*

CD or certificate of deposit: Nope, there's no music on this CD. This one is a secure investment of money that can yield more than an ordinary bank account. You must keep your money in it for the given amount of time on the certificate: 3 months, 6 months, 1 year, etc., in order to accrue the interest that particular CD promised. A 1 year CD yields a higher percentage of interest than a 3 month CD.

But don't tie up exorbitant amounts of your parent's money in CDs and be sure you open them within the given time period, when they come due, or they will be locked up for another stint of time and you'll have to wait to get at your money. Your parent's **financial planner** can help you find the best ways to have some **liquid assets** available while keeping your parent in a long-term investment that can keep up with inflation.

Contingent Beneficiaries: see **Secondary beneficiaries**

DOW: The DOW means, Dow Jones Industrial Average. It is one of the daily indicators of how our economy is doing. The DOW is made up of 30 companies which represent our Gross National Product (GNP). If the bulk of the companies in the DOW group do well, the DOW numbers will go up. The highest the DOW averages have read as of 2010 was 14,000 in the summer of 2007. However, in the early part of 2009, the DOW was under 7000. So you can see that it can fluctuate a lot and thus your parent's investments can soar or be greatly reduced. So try to diversify their money: bonds, treasuries, precious metals, property . . . as well as stocks.

Durable Power of Attorney or POA: The POA is usually the title given to one of the children of your parents. This is an *official* title with *official* papers to validate it. In fact, there are TWO Power of Attorney responsibilities. One is over your parent's **health** and the other is over your parent's **finances**. Your parent will want TWO papers drawn up to designate the person in charge of these two areas.

If you are the POA over your parent's finances, be sure you keep good receipts and records. And keep visiting your parent to reassure them you aren't misusing your powers and that you do care about them. You may be POA for 5, 10, or 20 years. However, the power of the POA ends after your parent dies—that's when the **executor's** or **fiduciary's** duties begin.

Estate taxes: Each year, of course, your parent will have to file a Federal Tax Return. But the *Federal Estate Tax* is a different tax. It won't even be in question until after the death of your parent. And unless your parent's taxable estate (homes, joint tenancy property, etc.) is over a set amount established by the Federal Estate Tax law, you probably won't even have to be concerned about Federal Estate Taxes. *However, do consult with your parent's estate lawyer and financial advisor BEFORE your parent dies, because they may have suggestions on how to reduce that responsibility.* Also check for the inheritance taxes or estate taxes for the *state* that your parent resides in.

Executor (Executrix) or Personal Representative: Executor (the guy) or Executrix (the girl) is the person who is legally noted in the will of your parent to distribute the estate. In essence, if you are the executor, you're in charge of the estate after the death of your parent. Your POA title no longer has any powers once your parent dies—that's when the executor's duties begin.

Funeral Policy or Final Expense Policy: This is an insurance policy that can be purchased from a reputable insurance company for the purpose of paying for your parent's funeral. It takes the place of a prepaid funeral plan with the funeral home.

Fiduciary: Also called a **trustee.** This is a person, or it could be a bank, who is entrusted with the distribution of your parent's important stuff (money, possessions and such) upon the death of the one holding the **trust** (that would be your parent), according to the conditions of the trust. Which means you are probably named the fiduciary of your parent's trust (if they have one) and that means you need to know exactly what those conditions are. A fiduciary of a trust carries more responsibility than an **executor** of a **will**. Talk to the estate lawyer about the extended responsibility.

Funds: Funds are a group of investments under a variety of headings, such as, aggressive growth funds, **income funds, bond funds**, etc. When these investment funds are grouped together into a **mutual fund**, they are known as a "family." With so many funds and so little time, you may want to trust your parent's financial planner to select what is right for your parent's situation.

Geriatric Care Manager: If you are having trouble finding the appropriate care assessment for your parent, needing screening and monitoring of in-home help, wanting to review the financial, legal and medical issues for your parent and need all around counseling and support in your eldercare decisions, you may want to look into a professional **geriatric care manager**. This person can be especially helpful if you are trying to be a long distance caregiver. Check out the specific duties and how to locate one near you through the **National Association of Professional Geriatric Care Managers** NAPGCM at **www.caremanager.org**

Gifting: Who wouldn't like a gift? Well, this gifting from your parent's **IRA** or investments must be done with the consent of the living parent and within the laws of your state. It may insure that a large estate does not incur exorbitant taxes after the death of the parent by gifting some of the estate to the heirs before your parent passes away.

If your parent has a large estate and they want to give some of the estate to their children, while they are still alive, they can.

Do be careful that it does not jeopardize your parent's future care or be outside of the legal gifting limits of the law. Consult with your parent's financial advisor, estate lawyer, care facility and doctor before considering this option.

Inflation: You'll hear this term a lot when you invest your parent's money. It refers to the cost of living that inevitably goes up, a lot or a little, about 3-6% per year. But one thing's for sure, it always goes up. Just look back on your own lifetime. Next to over-spending, inflation is the biggest threat to your parent's future.

EXAMPLE: A new car in the early seventies cost about $3000. A new car in the early 21st century cost about $25,000. That's inflation. And since your parent is probably retired and living off a fixed income (Social Security and/ or IRA withdrawals), their income won't go up with inflation and their next doctor appointment or car may be too expensive for their budget.

Investing their money wisely could help them "hedge" inflation, which simply stated means that they can keep up with inflation or even stay ahead of it.

Inheritance Taxes: Inheritance tax is also known as estate tax. It's a tax that may be due after the death of your parent, depending on the size of their estate. Small estates, life insurance policies, some annuities and less valuable personal possessions aren't taxable.

Responsible **gifting** of your parent's estate, before they die, could be a way to avoid high taxes on a large estate. Check with an estate lawyer and financial advisor and be sure to calculate senior facility costs and any future perceived medical needs into your decision.

INSURANCE: Insurance is a policy that will pay you when bad things happen. A good policy can help pay for hospital stays, car accidents, house or apartment disasters and even pay out an immediate income, after your parent dies.

You do want to be sure your parent has the following insurances:
1. Homeowners or Rental, *if they're in a house, condo, or apartment, but probably not assisted living or nursing home.*
2. Auto, *if they are still driving.*
3. Health, *which may be under Group from previous employment, Medigap, Medicare and Medicare supplement.*
4. Long Term Care, *if they are 80 or younger and can get reasonable coverage.*
5. Your parent may or may not need Life insurance.

- **Insurance Premiums:** This is the monthly payment you make to your insurance company to continue your agreed upon coverage.

- **Secondary Insurance:** When Medicare tells you what they won't pay, that's when you want to turn the bill over to a secondary insurance coverage. Your parent may have a secondary insurance with the company they worked for or they may have it with an insurance company or a **Medigap** policy. Check it out. Also, consider dental, optical, and hearing aid insurance, if you can get it, because **Medicare** doesn't cover any of these.

- **Term Life Insurance:** This is the most straightforward and often least expensive life insurance for the coverage. However, term life may be too costly due to the age of your parent. If your parent dies in a certain time period, their beneficiaries collect the amount that your parent was insured for. If they live after that agreed upon term, the beneficiaries get nothing and the policy ends with NO cash value.

  While a term life policy could be good for a short period, especially for a younger parent with a mortgage and children to put through college, it doesn't accumulate money to borrow against and may not be good for a senior parent.

- **Primary Insurance:** This is the first insurance card that you take out of your wallet because it is the one designated to pay most of the cost of your medical bills. For your parent, that should be **Medicare** or a **Medicare Advantage** program or, if they are eligible for **Medcaid**, then Medicaid would be their primary insurance.

- **Umbrella Insurance:** No, this isn't an insurance for umbrellas but it does offer your parent a great coverage in the case of a law suit over a car wreck or accident in their home or business. There are two categories under this particular insurance policy: *personal* (for the car and home) and *commercial* (for the business).

  With frivolous law suits running rampant today, it's comforting to know that your parent can get up to $2,000,000 worth of extra coverage (in addition to their home and car insurance) to cover any law suits against your parent. For just a few hundred dollars a year, it could save your parent's estate and your inheritance.

- **Universal Life Insurance:** This policy combines a death benefit with **tax-deferred** savings.

  You can increase or decrease the amount of the policy while it is in force. You can take out money from the savings portion and still have a death benefit for your beneficiaries who will owe no tax on the amount paid. You do pay for this flexibility with higher fees and administrative costs.

- **Variable Life Insurance:** This is a form of cash-value insurance designed for investing. You can decide where you want to invest your cash value. The value of your policy will be determined by how you were invested. It can go up or down.

- **Whole Life Insurance:** Whole life is sometimes called "Straight Life". This is a more traditional life insurance policy. The **premiums** stay the same for the life of the policy. Once you pay all the premiums, the policy stays in effect until you die. Your money does accumulate a cash reserve, which you can borrow on but you have no control over the way that it's invested.

Investments: see **Funds**

IRA: Individual Retirement Account: Not to be confused with the IRS (Internal Revenue Service that collects income tax each year), the **IRA** is a tax-deferred investment package that you can roll your parent's 401K, 403B, or 457 into. It allows your parent to control how they want to invest their money, rather than accepting the investment package that their company has chosen. That word, "**rollover**" is very important. Discuss **rollover** plans with your parent's financial advisor before accepting any checks from your parent's retirement plan.

IRS: Internal Revenue Service: If you're like me and trip over all the initials we use to describe various businesses and services, I just thought I would clarify that IRS is not an IRA. You pay your taxes to the IRS every April 15th and you hopefully are making money from your IRA.

Joint Account: If both parents are still alive and married to each other, they probably have a joint account. A joint account on their checking and savings simply means that either one of the people named on that account can withdraw money from the checking or saving accounts.

If either or both of your parents are having a bit of a struggle physically or mentally, it may be a good idea for you, their **POA**, to be added to their joint account. You would be listed under your parent with the added prefix of "**POA**". What that means is you would have access to your parent's saving and checking account, while you are POA, but your parent would be the one to declare any interest gains on their tax return.

You will need to keep receipts and make notations in the checkbook, in order to qualify the expenditures as being used for your parent. While you would have access to the money, as POA, you can't frivolously use the money for yourself. It's kind of a check and balance system to cut down on the greed factor. It's especially beneficial if your parent is incompetent or lives in another city.

After your parent dies, the **executor** needs access to the money to pay outstanding bills. Without a joint account between you and your parent, the bank could "freeze" the account and you will have to wait until the will comes out of probate to pay the bills.

Remember, the money is not yours until the will is settled and all bills are paid; it is a part of your parent's estate and therefore any remaining sum should be evenly distributed amongst the heirs.

Joint Tenants with right of survivorship: When a single property is jointly owned by two or more persons (not necessarily related), under one title, with equal rights to the property—upon the death of one of the joint tenants, the property automatically transfers to the surviving tenant. In other words, if your parent has a business partner, don't assume that the business will be a part of your parent's estate when they die. It may go to the business partner. Read over all contracts carefully.

Liquid assets: This is a term used to describe an **asset** that you can liquidate immediately, when you need the cash. Obviously, hard cash in your parent's wallet, in the cookie jar or under their mattress would be a liquid asset. Cash in a checking and savings account would also be considered liquid assets—because you can get the money within a few minutes or a day or two.

However, **CD**s, cars, houses, silver bouillons, jewelry and collectables are NOT "liquid". They may have a lot of value, but you have to sell them first. And that could take months. You always want to have a reasonable about of liquid assets for such things as medical equipment, general doctor bills and repairs that may arise. Check with your parent's financial advisor and doctor for an appropriate amount to have on hand—possibly $10,000 to $15,000.

Long-term care: Due to incredible life-saving emergency care, surgical advances and new medications, we are living longer than our forefathers. It's not uncommon to hear of someone living well into their 90s.

On the downside, we also have a rise in the cost of the health care facilities for our aging population. Because there is a good chance that your parent will need in-home nursing care, assisted living or nursing home care, and because most insurance policies only pay for hospitals but not long-term care facilities, it's good to look into a long-term care policy. You can check it out with your insurance agent or financial planner. If your parent qualifies, they can get a policy started, even when they are 80.

Mutual Funds: There are lots of different mutual funds out there. And your financial planner will have several mutual funds to offer you through his company. These mutual funds are "managed", meaning that someone will be checking on your parent's funds and moving their money around within the mutual fund as the economy dictates.

Your planner may want to invest your parent's money in some **moderate to low-risk funds**, according to your parent's age and comfort level with these types of investments. Check the "track record" of the mutual fund for at least the last 30 years.

Mutual funds allow you to invest in a wide variety of funds such as: **aggressive growth funds, growth and income funds, small company growth funds, balanced funds, option income funds, international stock and bond funds, global funds, bond funds, high yield funds**, and **tax-free high yield funds.**

Be careful about high-risk funds for your aging parent's investments. A good fund should be able to yield an average 6% to 7% interest on your parent's investment annually. So the idea is to not take out more than 6% or 7% a year for living expenses. If your parent is in their late eighties or early nineties, has a terminal health condition and a large investment, you may decide to take out more from their investment. Check with your parent's **financial planner** and **CPA** to be sure of how it will effect their investment and any income tax increase due to withdrawals.

POA (Power of Attorney) or Durable Power of Attorney: Check under "**Durable Power of Attorney.**"

POD: Payable on Death See TOD

Prepaid Funeral: This is a contract that your parent completes with the funeral home of your parent's choice. The funeral home should be able to take care of all the details that your parent desires for their funeral because of the specific wording of the prepaid funeral contract.

Needless to say, this can lift a burden off you, the bereaving caregiver, when the time comes and it assures your parent that their wishes will be carried out.

Because it is prepaid, you won't have to worry about having enough money for the funeral expenses and it can save money, since you pay at today's prices for a funeral that may not take place for ten or more years. *(There may be some minor expenses that you did not have in the prepaid funeral, such as extra cost of transporting the body from another town, raised cost of florist's fees, etc. but it shouldn't cost more than a few hundred dollars, as opposed to over $7000 for a 2011 funeral.)*

*(Also check out chapter 7 and your insurance agent for a **Final Expense Policy** that covers funeral expenses.)*

Preplanned Funeral: Unlike the prepaid funeral, this is just a record that you would keep that describes everything your parent would like to have done at their funeral. Where they want to be buried, how they would like the funeral to be run, any organizations they may want recognized through donations, etc. *(A more complete list of items to consider for funerals can be found in chapters 7 and 14.)*

Portfolio: This is a term that is used to describe all of your parent's investments; stocks, bonds, savings, CDs, etc. Your parent's financial portfolio is an overview of what they are worth. It's usually safer to have a diversified portfolio. In other words, don't put all your parent's eggs (money) in one basket (investment).

Premiums: This is what insurance companies call the money you owe them. You can pay your insurance premiums monthly, quarterly, or annually.

Retirement Account: One type of this tax-deferred sum of money, which is now nearly extinct, is called a pension and it is given to your parent by their company upon their retirement. The more recent forms of retirement accounts are paid for by the employee and the company will often match a portion of the amount the employee pays into it. These retirement accounts are called by different names like **401Ks** or **403Bs**. They are invested. And the good news is that the retired person, namely your parent, doesn't owe any taxes on this investment earning until they take the money out of the account.

A 401K can be **rolled over** into an **IRA** and invested into a mutual fund, annuity, or any number of investment opportunities. If you don't roll it over into a tax-deferred investment and cash it out, you will owe taxes on its entire value (which could be 100's of thousands of dollars). So check with your financial advisor before making a decision for your retirement account and be sure you **roll it over** into their investment package to avoid taxes.

Rollover: This is an investment term that describes how a person is to transfer one retirement investment into another. It is a way of protecting the funds from being taxed until your parent removes the money from the account, often withdrawing small monthly sums as an income. Be sure you check with your parent's financial advisor to be sure their retirement accounts are properly distributed via rollovers.

Secondary Insurance: See **INSURANCE: Secondary Insurance**

Secondary beneficiaries: Your parent's Will, insurance policy and investments should list their spouse as the primary beneficiary, unless their spouse died or they are divorced. But these important papers should also list the **secondary beneficiaries** also called the **contingent beneficiaries** (usually the children) in what is known as a **TOD** clause. *(Note the Survivorships and Beneficiary's chart in chapter 2)*

SEP: Simplified Employee Pension plan: An SEP plan allows employers to contribute to traditional IRAs (SEP-IRAs) set up for employees. With this pension plan, any size business, even a self-employed business, can establish an SEP.

Social Security: There is a lot of talk about whether Social Security will still be around in the next thirty or forty years. I don't know. But it is still intact as of the writing of this book. And your parent has probably put money into it out of their paychecks when they were working so they don't have to feel that this is a government handout.

When your parent reaches 65 years of age, your parent is entitled to a set amount of monthly income, based on how much they earned when they worked, how long they worked and if they are married. Your parent can claim their Social Security benefits as early as 62, but they will receive a slightly reduced amount.

Check with the Social Security Office nearest you to apply at least a month before your 62nd, 65th or 67th birthday, depending on when you are going to take distributions so that your benefits will start right away. (If you apply too early, they won't process your application.) Bring a photo ID and your birth certificate when you apply. You actually get your first check one month after your birthday.

Stocks: This signifies ownership in a company that your parent purchases, via shares, from a corporation or they may purchase it within their mutual fund and only see it listed on the investment company's monthly report. In essence, by buying a stock in a company, your parent will own a piece (albeit a small piece) of that company.

If the company does well, your parent makes money. If the company does poorly or goes bankrupt, or the CEO bails out with a golden parachute, your parent's stocks could be greatly reduced or worthless.

Unlike **CD**s and some **bonds**, there is no guarantee that your parent will even retain the original value of the stock. Stocks are more volatile. In other words, your parent can make a lot of money with stocks in a **bull market** but they can also lose a lot in a **bear market**. And with an aging parent, you want to be careful that they don't risk their money on any "get rich quick" stocks.

Talk to your parent's financial planner. Try to get your parent's **portfolio** diversified with solid stocks in a variety of areas and even various parts of the world.

Survivorship Will: It's a simple Will between a husband and wife. If one dies, the other gets everything. Also, be sure they have **secondary** (or **contingent**) **beneficiaries** (usually their children). (*Note chapter 2*)

TAXES: Federal Estate Taxes: see **Estate Taxes**

- **State Inheritance Taxes:** Even if your parent's estate is not subject to Federal Estate Taxes, it still may incur State Inheritance Taxes. So check with your parent's estate lawyer and financial advisor.

Tax-deferred: This is a term used for certain investments and insurances. It means that your parent doesn't have to pay tax on the interest earned in a "tax-deferred investment." Your parent only pays taxes when they take the money out of the investment. (Let's say your parent earned $100,000 on their IRA investments this year but only took $25,000 out of their IRA for living expenses. They would only owe taxes on the $25,000 withdrawal, if that's applicable.)

Tax Shelter: This is a term used to describe a legal method of minimizing or decreasing an investor's taxable income, also known as **tax-deferred** but not to be confused with *tax evasion*. While you don't owe any taxes on the IRA while it is earning money for you in the account, you may owe taxes when you take out that money, depending on your age and the amount of the withdrawal. That's where your financial advisor and CPA come in. Consult with them before doing any withdrawals.

TOD—Transfer on Death or POD—Payable on Death: This is an important clause to add to any investments, savings or insurance policies that your parent might have. It makes distribution of your parent's inheritance, after their death, a lot easier with less feuding between the heirs and if all financial papers have a TOD clause, you may be able to avoid **probate**. *(Check with the estate lawyer.)*

The way a TOD works is this: after your parent's death, when you have produced a death certificate to the investment and/or insurance company, that company will notify the heirs listed in the TOD clause of each investment and the amount in the account on the day of your parent's death.

The heirs listed on the investments will then be asked to sign papers designating if they want to cash out the investment or continue holding onto it. If they cash out, a check will be sent to them; if they remain invested, they will become owners of that portion of the investment and they can continue to receive notices of the progress of their investment.

Personally, I have found it cleans up the bookkeeping to just cash out but that is up to you and your heirs and your financial advisor.

Trust: A Trust is like an elaborate last will and testament, the big difference is that a trust can keep any property and assets out of **probate**, which can be time consuming and costly. The reason it avoids probate is that your parent will have transferred all their property, assets, bank accounts, securities and real estate to a person they "Trust" who is called the **trustee**—hence the name. And usually a Trust is set up for larger estates of $500,000 or more.

If your parent chooses a Trust, they will be able to have their estate managed by a **trustee** before and/or after their death—which is the difference between a **Living Trust** (effective while they're alive) and a **Testamentary Trust** (effective after they die).

A Trust may allow a parent to know that their inheritance will be uniquely distributed in small increments to pay for a grandchild's college or to be given to a charity or to run a business. A Trust costs more than a Will to prepare but it may be preferred due to the size of an estate or specific desires of your parent.

Trustee: see **Fiduciary**

Will or Last Will and Testament: This can be a simple or complex legal document that names the **executor** of your parent's estate, who will receive your parent's **estate**, who will serve as **guardian** of your parent's children or pets (if that applies), and any other specific provisions.

A simple Will normally cost less than a hundred dollars to create or you can buy a kit of documents from an office supply store that will allow you to create your own Will, living will and POA papers.

Prepaid Legal Services will create a Will for you as well as give you other monthly legal advice. *Suze Orman* has an entire portfolio of 50 documents to create off your computer. *(Note sources in chapter 15)*

However, for more precise features, specific to your parent's needs, an estate lawyer is probably your best way to go. Do remember that the more elaborate the will, the more expensive the bill. If the estate is large or complicated, you may want to ask the estate lawyer about drawing up a **trust** instead.

*(By the way, do not include your parent's funeral wishes in a Will, since the Will is usually read **after** the funeral. Instead, make arrangements with the funeral home as a preplanned or prepaid funeral or have them designate their wishes to the family in writing. Check out chapter 15.)*

❷ Medical Terms

Advanced directives: This is the term given to legal documents pertaining to the medical care of your parent. Their **living will** and **DNR** papers would come under this heading.

Alzheimer's disease and dementia: Both ailments have very similar resultant behaviors but the main difference is how they began or are progressing.

One form of dementia, *Alzheimer's disease*, is a disease of the brain that actually alters its composition. Brain cells are essentially being destroyed. Alzheimer's has been linked to the lack of brain use, such as excessive TV watching or very little reading, ingestion of Aluminum through cookware or canned foods and inheritance. No one knows for sure. There are medications, such as Aricept, that are helping patients inhibit the brain cell loss for Alzheimer's patients and it has been beneficial for other forms of dementia and even stroke patients, so prompt and accurate diagnosis is important. And you may have to seek a **geriatric psychologist** to properly assess your parent.

*You may want to read my book, **Inside Mom's Mind**, for a walk into the life of my Alzheimer's mother and her caregiver—that's me. It helps you to know the thoughts of the Alzheimer's patient, while helping to encourage the caregiver. The book has over 100 ideas for making the journey into forgetfulness a little more pleasant. Check it out on my web page, www.donnatrickett.com or to learn more about Alzheimer's go to www.alz.org (the Alzheimer's Association website)*

Assisted Living: This is a housing option for someone who may require assistance each day with getting dressed, bathed, eating right and remembering to take their medications. While this may seem like a nursing home because there is usually only one room and a bath with no kitchen, assisted living is very different. First of all it is cheaper than a nursing home, it gives the patient more freedom to move freely around the building or campus surrounding the facility and the patients are more conversant and mobile than in a nursing home. Also, there are fewer registered nurses on duty in assisted living because the patients do not require round-the-clock nursing care.

Caregiver: Caregiver is a generic term that simply means, "one who cares for another". It could refer to a nurse, adult child, concerned friend or staff member in a nursing home. You may be considered your parent's caregiver because they need you but if you are not legally pronounced their **POA** over their health and finances, you may be incapable of helping them in the more crucial areas.

Chronically ill: If you, the caregiver, are seeking financial assistance for your parent through Medicare, Medicaid or a Federal Income Tax deduction, you will need documentation by a licensed health care practitioner that states your parent is chronically ill.

Death certificate: This is an official document declaring the actual date, cause and place of death. You will need several originals to give to the bank, Social Security office, investment agencies, insurance agents, etc. They can be ordered by the funeral home before the funeral or you can acquire them from the health agency's vital statistics department in the county where your parent died. This little piece of paper can cost between $2 and $20, depending on what state your parent died in. And you may need as many as 10 certificates to close up the entire estate.

DNR or Do Not Resuscitate orders: Even though your parent may have expressed their wishes in their **living will,** to not be kept on life support, that is NOT the same as DNR. DNR papers are drawn up by the doctor to announce to any other doctor or emergency team that they should not try to resuscitate your parent with mouth to mouth, chest compressions, paddles, etc. However, as in most medical procedures, it gets a little more complicated than that. That's because there are TWO kinds of Do Not Resuscitate options. DNR-cc and DNR-arrest Let's look at the first one.

- **DNR-cc (do not resuscitate, comfort care only)** means you don't want your parent operated on, tested, given any shots or IVs for the purpose of sustaining their life, unless the doctor first talks to you, your parent's POA over their health. Your parent should be made comfortable and allowed to enjoy their last days in a comfortable setting at home, if you can provide that, or in a restful room at their facility. If you are going to work with **hospice,** you will need to have DNR-cc papers.

Always have a copy of the DNR papers on your person when you take your parent on a trip, to the hospital, a new housing establishment and in the hands of any healthcare providers. *(For more understanding of why you need DNR papers, read over chapter 4)*

- **DNR-arrest or Do Not Resuscitate—Arrest Orders:** DNR-arrest papers are when your parent may go into a medical facility and then complications may arise that requires added testing or medications. You are granting the physician the right to commit to further testing and medications as he considers necessary to prolong their life but you don't want the medical personnel to resuscitate your parent if your parent should go into cardiac arrest during these treatments.

The **POA** does not have to be consulted in this case. A doctor can quickly continue treatment and testing, as he sees fit. Doctors prefer DNR-arrest because they don't have to stop in the middle of their treatment to call the POA.

The difference between DNR-cc and DNR-arrest is really a matter of how much you want to be involved in the decisions over your parent's health. If you know that your parent does not want a lot of surgeries, experimental drugs, or prolonged hospital stays or is just getting too old to endure these procedures—then DNR-cc is most likely the better choice. But if you're uncomfortable with this decision or you just don't want to get called all the time by the doctors and nurses about procedures you don't understand, the DNR-arrest order is probably a better choice for you. Discuss it with your parent, *if they are able to rationally consider such decisions,* your siblings, your parent's doctor, the head nurse at the facility or your parent's hospice nurse, *if you are working with them.*

DNR options may change as your parent's condition changes, so be alert to your parent's wishes and their particular health situation.

Always have a copy of the DNR papers on your person, when you take your parent on a trip, to the hospital, a new housing establishment, and any healthcare providers. *(For more understanding of why you need DNR papers, read over chapter 4)*

Durable Power of Attorney over Health or POA: POA is usually the title given to one of the children of your parents. This is an "official" title with "official" papers to validate the fact. Also, there are TWO Power of Attorney responsibilities. One is **POA over your parent's health** and another is **POA over your parent's finances.** Your parent will want TWO papers drawn up to designate the person in charge of these two distinct areas.

Durable Power of Attorney over their health is a very powerful title. The person holding this paper is in charge of a big piece of their elderly parent's health and thus a chunk of their life. Keep in touch with the doctor or nurse practitioner and the head nurse so you can make an educated decision. And do understand that "plugs" are not "pulled" without the decision and agreement of the attending physician. So you do have some checks and balances over the really awesome decisions. Plus it's always a good idea to keep up communications about your parent's state of health with any siblings or other close relatives. It will help them to understand what you are going through and allow them to voice their opinion while taking some of the weight off your shoulders.

Geriatric Care Manager: If you are having trouble finding the appropriate care assessment for your parent, needing screening and monitoring of in-home help, wanting to review the financial, legal and medical issues for your parent and need all around counseling and support in your eldercare decisions, you may want to look into a professional **geriatric care manager.** This person can be especially helpful if you are trying to be a long distance caregiver. Check out the specific duties and how to locate one near you through the **National Association of Professional Geriatric Care Managers** NAPGCM at **www.caremanager.org**

Geriatric Psychologist: You are probably familiar with the term *psychologist* but you may confuse that term with a *psychiatrist.* And then there is the *geriatric* part of this doctor's title. So let me explain. First of all, a *psychiatrist* is a medical doctor who uses psychotherapy, may prescribe medications, and may even perform electroconvulsive therapy. A *psychologist,* on the other hand, is NOT a medical doctor but he may hold a PhD. A *psychologist* primarily aids their patient by counseling and psychotherapy.

Now let's add *geriatric* to the mix and we have a psychologist who focuses on the health care of the *elderly.* This is the person who can help you discover the mental status of your dementia parent. That's important because the sooner you discover if your parent has Alzheimer's, or another form of dementia, the sooner you can start them on a medication that may slow down the acceleration of the disease for a few years. So don't be afraid to have your parent tested but you will need to get any medication prescriptions from a medical doctor.

Why not use a medical doctor in the first place? Because most medical doctors don't have the time or skills to analyze the subtle difference between an Alzheimer's senior patient and just a matter of forgetfulness that is seen in most aging patients. Also, ordinary psychologists are not trained in that unique area of senior care. You will find that a **geriatric psychologist** *can direct you to a more exact understanding of your parent's forgetful condition.*

Hospice: This group of caring individuals has supplied physical, emotional, and spiritual support to millions of people during the difficulty of caring for a critically ill loved one. Their help is free. They're paid for by **Medicare** and private donations.

Hospice usually pays for medications and equipment used for comfort care. They will attend to the patient and the caregivers at any hour and they can add devotional care, if you ask. Don't hesitate to call them, even if you're not sure your parent qualifies.

Living Will: The living will, or **physician's directive**, has nothing to do with the last will and testament that bequeaths (gives) the estate to the heirs (persons that inherit everything).

The **living will** deals with the wishes of your parent about their health care under critical conditions. Specifically, the living will lets the caregiver and doctors know what your parent would want done if they were to find themselves in a situation where they were alive but unable to speak. It specifies what to do about life support systems. As **POA** over their health, it's important that you acknowledge and agree to carry out your parent's wishes in their living will.

Be sure the facility that is housing your parent; whether it's a nursing home, retirement community or hospital; has a copy of this document.

Long-term care: Because it's likely that your parent will need in-home nursing care, assisted living or nursing home care sometime in their life and because most insurances only pay for hospital stays and short stays for rehabilitation in nursing home facilities, it's good to look into a long-term care policy.

Long-term care policies will pay a monthly agreed upon amount for skilled nursing care in assisted living facilities and nursing homes. Some policies will even pay for in-home nursing care and your parent will probably find the policy increasing to match inflation. They can be difficult or expensive to buy, but if your parent is 80 or younger, they may be eligible, and the policy could be beneficial. You can check it out with your insurance agent and/or financial planner.

Medicaid: Medicaid is a federally funded medical assistance coverage for those individuals at a low-income level. **Medicare** helps pay for medical care for most people 65 and over but if that individual should run out of their savings and assets due to health problems or an economic downturn, **Medicaid** will step in under certain parameters*.

Often when a patient is put into the Medicaid category, they are moved to a Medicaid-approved facility and may need to change doctors.

Do understand that Medicaid will not pay if your parent had gifted away or carelessly spent large sums of money within 5 years or more of their financial bankruptcy. So be responsible as their POA over their finances and check out the requirements with www.medicaid.com or your doctor.

Medicare (Medicare Part A and B): Medicare is a limited medical coverage for persons 65 or over. It becomes your parent's primary insurance but, if you want to reduce your medical costs still more, you need a Medicare supplemental or Medicare advantage plan for the parts that are not covered by Medicare alone.

The entitlement coverage for seniors is **Medicare Part A.** To get more coverage, which you really do need, then sign up for **Medicare Part B,** as well. *(Check out chapter 5.)*

Medicare Advantage (Medicare Part C): With Medicare Advantage you can be covered with everything Medicare Part A and B cover and have some benefits included that are not in Medicare Part A and B, like a prescription drug discount plan and Silver Sneakers. Medicare Part C plans may or may not require extra monthly fees. And they do require the patient going to accepted doctors and hospitals in the plan. Before acquiring Medicare Advantage plan you must sign up for Medicare Part A and B.

When you fill out a medical form, Medicare Advantage is your primary insurance. (But, again, don't get rid of your Medicare card, put it in a safe place.)

Medicare supplement (Medigap): Medicare does not cover the first several days in the hospital, nor do they cover prescription drugs, specialists or many hospital tests and procedures. To feel more at peace with the threat of old age and the inevitable surgeries that seem to follow the Medicare crowd, it does pay to look into a **Medicare supplemental insurance** (also known as **Medigap**).

Various letters in the alphabet list these supplemental policies. All the **A, B, C,** etc. coverages give the same benefits, no matter which provider you choose. In other words an **A** supplemental policy with one company will cover the exact same things that the **A** supplemental policy covers with another company. The only thing that varies is the price and the reputation of the company that offers it, so shop around.

While Medicare coverage payments are automatically withdrawn from your Social Security check, the supplemental plans do add an additional monthly fee. But you should be able to use any doctor or hospital that accepts Medicare. *(LOTS more info in chapter 5.)*

Medigap: See Medicare supplement

Nursing Home: Normally your parent will not be placed in a nursing home unless they require round the clock skilled nursing care. If they only need help in remembering their medications, getting dressed or having hot meals, consider **Assisted Living** or Residential Care.

And if you are expecting Medicare to pay for a nursing home, your parent will have to spend a specific amount of days and nights in a hospital first and be assigned to the nursing home by the attending physician. (Check Medicare's requirements) After that, Medicaid may come on the scene to pay for the nursing home but your parent needs to meet their low-income requirements and "look back" policy . . . so check it out on their websites www.medicaid.com and www.medicare.com

Physician's Directive: See **Living Will**

POA (Power of Attorney) or Durable Power of Attorney over Health: Check under "**Durable Power of Attorney**".

Prepaid Funeral: This is a contract that your parent completes with the funeral home of your parent's choice. The funeral home should be able to take care of all the details that your parent desires for their funeral because of the specific wording of the prepaid funeral contract.

The funeral home should:
   (1) Notify the newspaper/newspapers.
   (2) Order the family bouquets.
   (3) Have the appropriate coffin and funeral attire ready (if you've left them the clothes you want for your parent).
   (4) Order the **death certificates.**
   (5) Arrange for the music of your parent's choice.
   (6) If your parent chose cremation, they will place their ashes in requested urn in a tasteful setting.
   (7) Have pictures or memorabilia on display at the viewing and funeral (if you've left pictures with them ahead of time).

Because it is prepaid, you won't have to worry about having enough money for the funeral expenses and it can save money, since you pay at today's prices for a funeral that may not take place for ten or more years. *(There may be some minor expenses that you did not have in the prepaid funeral, such as extra cost of transporting the body from another town, increased cost of florist's fees, etc. but it shouldn't cost more than a few hundred dollars, as opposed to over $7000 for a 2011 funeral.)*

Check on the reputability of the funeral home and the way that they are investing your parent's money. It should be in a **trust.** Talk to your financial planner and several funeral directors before finalizing your decision. If your parent has a good investment portfolio, you may not want the pre-paid funeral but you should record their desire for the way they wish their funeral to be conducted. Assure your parent you will carry out their wishes.

*(Also check with your insurance agent for a **Final Expense Policy** that covers funeral expenses.)*

Preplanned Funeral: Unlike the prepaid funeral, this is just a record that you would keep that describes everything your parent would like to have done at their funeral. Where they want to be buried, how they would like the funeral to be run and any organizations they may want to be recognized through donations, etc. Do not include funeral plans in the Will since the Will is not read until AFTER the funeral. *(A more complete list of items for funerals can be found in chapter 14.)*

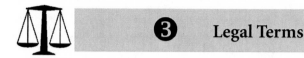

3 Legal Terms

Beneficiaries or heirs: That's the name given to someone who benefits, in money or things, from the death of someone else. In other words, if you're named as a beneficiary in your parent's life insurance policy, investment distribution, will, or trust, then you're the heir due to receive the asset. There may be more than one beneficiary or heir, especially if your parent has more than one child. But beneficiaries can be grandchildren, churches, nonprofit organizations, a friend, or yes, even a pet. [There are **primary beneficiaries** (such as the spouse) and **secondary beneficiaries** (also known as **contingent beneficiaries**), usually the children or grandchildren.] *(Note chart in chapter 2)*

Bequest: A legal term that simply means the act of giving or passing on to another. The Will could read, "I leave everything to my husband," but instead it reads, "I bequest everything to my husband." It sounds more official.

Codicil: Rather than rewriting a new Will whenever your parent wants to change something, they can simply ask the estate lawyer to add a codicil. It's like an amendment to the constitution. It just adds one point, like a change in the executor or an addition to the heirs.

Conservator: This is an individual (a **guardian**) who is appointed by the court to supervise another person or that person's financial affairs. A conservatorship is created in order to ensure that a mentally or physically challenged individual gets good care and their money will not be recklessly spent.

Custodian or Guardian: This is the person appointed to care for an individual that is designated by the courts in a custodianship or guardianship. See Custodianship below.

Custodianship or Guardianship: If your parent is still in charge of a minor child or if they have had to take care of a mentally or physically challenged adult child, they need to designate, in their **will** or **trust**, a guardian or custodian for that child.

These terms may also apply to you, the executor of your parent's Will, if you've been given charge of a business, charity or estate after the death of your parent. Even your parent's pet can be assigned a guardian in their Will or trust.

In cases where the parent may be considered mentally incompetent, you may request to be their **guardian**, which means you are in charge of all the decisions for their money and health. Be very careful when officially designating yourself as guardian over your parent because it may be contested by the other heirs, which could get you into some legal hassles, plus it is a gigantic responsibility—much greater than being appointed POA because you'll be making *all* the decisions for your parent, as if they were your child.

Be sure to ask the attorney exactly what the duties of a guardian are before creating the official paperwork.

Durable Power of Attorney or POA: POA is usually the title given to one of the children of your parent. This is an "official" title with "official" papers to validate the fact. Also, there are TWO Power of Attorney responsibilities.

One is **POA over your parent's health** and another is **POA over your parent's finances.** Your parent will want TWO papers drawn up to designate the person in charge of these two distinct areas.

Make copies of these papers and give them to your parent's bank, hospital (if your parent is a patient), and nursing home, or other housing facility of your parent.

Durable Power of Attorney is a very powerful title. The person holding these papers is in charge of their elderly parent's health and money, and thus a chunk of their life. Be sure you keep receipts and records. And keep visiting your parent to reassure them you aren't misusing your powers. The power of the POA is voided after your parent dies, that's when the **executor's** duties kick in.

Estate: While an estate is often referred to as a large house and property, in the legal sense, it means anything that a person possesses, including their debts and any taxes due, after they die. Their house, car, boat, jewelry, bank accounts, IRA and investments are all a part of their estate.

Estate taxes: As the old saying goes, there are only two things we can count on in this life, death and taxes. This tax, also known as an inheritance tax, only applies after the death of your parent. The good news is, if the total amount of the estate does not exceed a set amount determined by the Federal government—you don't owe any Federal Estate Tax. However, you still may owe estate tax for the state they live in. Check with your parent's **estate lawyer**. Also check for the inheritance taxes or estate taxes in the state your parent resides.

Executor: The executor is the person who is named in the will and thus legally appointed to distribute the estate of your parent. (The executrix is the female counterpart.) In essence, the executor is in charge of the estate after the death of the parent. The POA no longer has any powers once your parent dies, that's when the executor's duties begin.

Fiduciary: See **Trustee.**

Geriatric Care Manager: If you are having trouble finding the appropriate care assessment for your parent, needing screening and monitoring of in-home help, wanting to review the financial, legal and medical issues for your parent and need all around counseling and support in your eldercare decisions, you may want to look into a professional **geriatric care manager**. This person can be especially helpful if you are trying to be a long distance caregiver. Check out the specific duties and how to locate one near you through the **National Association of Professional Geriatric Care Managers** NAPGCM at www.caremanager.org

Gifting: Who wouldn't like a gift? Well, this gifting must be done with the consent of the living parent and within the laws of your state. If your parent has a large estate and they want to give some of the estate to their children, while they are still alive, they can. Another benefit of gifting is the lowering of your parent's estate taxes after they die. In other words, more money stays in the family.

Gifting gives your parent a chance to see the joy their inheritance can bring through such gifts as paying for part of their grandchild's education or the down payment on a new home for their child. But be careful you keep to the rules of gifting and don't let your parent empty their account to where they can't afford good care in their golden years. Also, you don't want to jeopardize Medicaid benefits should they ever require that health care program. Check with their estate lawyer, health care provider and financial planner before considering this option.

Guardian: See **Custodian**

Heir: See **Beneficiaries**

Joint Tenants with right of survivorship: When a single property is jointly owned by two or more persons (not necessarily related), under one title, with equal rights to the property, upon the death of one of the joint tenants, the property automatically transfers to the surviving tenant. Therefore, it may not be a part of the inheritance of your parent's heirs.

Last Will and Testament: See **Will**

Living Will: The living will, or physician's directive, has nothing to do with the last will and testament that bequeaths (gives) the estate to the heirs (persons that inherit everything). The living will deals with the wishes of your parent about their healthcare under critical conditions.

Specifically, the living will lets the caregiver and doctors know what your parent would want done if they were still alive but unable to speak. It specifies what to do about life support systems. As **POA** over their health, it's important that you acknowledge and agree to carry out your parent's wishes in their living will and that you give copies to the hospital, nursing home or other place of residence of your parent.

Physician's Directive: Same as **Living Will.**

POA (Power of Attorney) or Durable Power of Attorney: See **Durable Power of Attorney**

POD: Payable on Death See TOD

Probate: This is the judicial determination of the validity of a **will**. Most people want to avoid probate because it can take a year or more to settle an estate after the death of someone and it may cost thousands of dollars in lawyer's fees. That's why many people look at creating a **trust**, because it can avoid probate.

A simple **will**, modest **estate**, and beneficiary clauses (*also known as TOD clause, transfer on death*) attached to all legal financial papers may also avoid probate.

So talk to your estate lawyer to see how you may be able to legally avoid probate for your parent's estate.

Testator: It's just a fancy legal term for the person who has a **will** drawn up for their estate. In your case, it would be your parent.

TOD—Transfer on Death or POD—Payable on Death: This is an important clause to add to any investments, savings, or insurance policies that your parent might have. It makes distribution of your parent's inheritance, after their death, a lot easier with less feuding between the heirs and if all financial papers have a TOD clause, you may be able to avoid probate. (Check with the estate lawyer)

The way a TOD works is this: after your parent's death, when you have produced a death certificate to the investment and/or insurance company, that company will notify the heirs listed in the TOD clause of each investment and the amount in the account on the day of your parent's death. The heirs listed on the investments will then be asked to sign papers designating if they want to cash out the investment or continue holding onto it. If they cash out, checks will be sent out; if they remain invested, they will become owners of that portion of the investment and they can continue to receive notices of the progress of their investment. Personally, I have found it cleans up the bookkeeping to just cash out but that is up to you and your heirs and your financial advisor.

Trust: A Trust is like an elaborate last will and testament, the big difference is that a trust can keep any property and assets out of **probate**, which can be time consuming and costly. The reason it avoids probate is that your parent will have transferred all their property, assets, bank accounts, securities and real estate to a person they "Trust" who is called the **trustee**—hence the name. And usually a Trust is set up for larger estates of $500,000 or more. If your parent chooses a trust, they will be able to have their estate managed by a **trustee** before and/or after their death—which is the difference between a Living Trust (effective while they're alive) and a Testamentary Trust (effective after they die). A Trust may allow a parent to know that their inheritance will be uniquely distributed in small increments to pay for a grandchild's college or to be given to a charity or to run a business. A Trust cost more than a Will to prepare but it may be preferred due to the size of an estate.

Trustee: A trustee (or **fiduciary**) is a person who is appointed to manage the trust that your parent may have set up. A Trustee may be necessary because the heirs of the trust are too young or not mentally or physically capable of taking care of themselves or the Trustee may be needed because the estate is so large and an existing business may be involved.

For whatever reasons your parent had for making a trust, the **trustee** could be one of your parent's children or a responsible bank, corporation or accounting individual who was preselected by your parent, much like the executor of the will.

Will or Last Will and Testament: This can be a simple or complex legal document that names the **executor** of your parent's estate, the heirs of your parent's **estate, guardians** of your parent's children or pets (if that applies) and any other specific provisions.

Wills normally cost less than a hundred dollars to create or you can buy a kit of documents from an office supply store that will allow you to create your own will, living will, and POA papers.

Prepaid Legal Services can create a Will for you as well as give you other monthly legal advice. Suze Orman has an entire portfolio of 50 documents to create off your computer. *(Note sources in chapter 15.)*

However, for more precise features, specific to your parent's needs, an estate lawyer is probably your best way to go. Do remember that the more elaborate the will, the more expensive the bill. If the estate is large or complicated, you may want to consider a **trust** instead of a will. Talk with the estate lawyer.

*(By the way, do not include your parent's funeral wishes in the Will, since the Will is usually read **after** the funeral. Instead, make arrangements with the funeral home as a preplanned or prepaid funeral or have them designate their wishes to the family in writing.)*

CHAPTER 9

HOUSING:
Where Should My Folks Live?

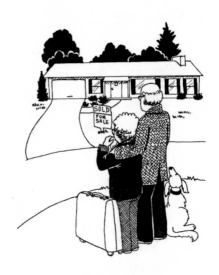

Your folks should continue to live wherever they like, as long as their health and finances will allow. The other day I was watching a reality TV show in which a senior adult had become obsessed with raising over one hundred cats inside her home. The ammonia smell was causing her lung problems; dead cats were found under her bed and behind boxes; and the family had stopped visiting her because of the smell. So I think, in some cases, there does need to be limits as to what is acceptable for your parent's housing choices. You may even need to seek psychological help and/or a professional organizer who can help them unclutter their home. It apparently can be a rather complicated situation but not an impossible one. Hopefully, you won't have to deal with the more severe issues of senior housing and instead they fall under one of the three categories I found in my caregiving experiences.

I've found that some seniors are able to climb a ladder to fix a gutter, get on their knees to scrub the floor and they seem to be able to manage their medications and diet without any help from outsiders, well into their eighties.

My mother-in-law, **Frances**, was just such a person. In fact, the activity kept her bones and muscles healthy and she slept better. Frances was able to stay in her home for over 50 years, 18 years after her husband died. She only required hospital and nursing home attention in the last few months of her life.

My father, **Donald**, on the other hand, went from strong to weak and back to healthy and back to weak again for a period of over ten years. His heart condition required various surgeries and drugs which kept him fluctuating in his health status. He occasionally needed around the clock attention, while at other times he was out tilling up their garden or doing the finishing touches on their add-on sunroom.

Thanks to my mother **Alice**'s active nature and over-all good health, she was able to care for my father during those bad times with a little help from a visiting nurse. After my Dad died, however, Mom began to drift into Alzheimer's and, despite her physical health; we had to consider other options for her care.

Which parent most resembles your parent's circumstances? Let's take a closer look at each individual's situation.

FRANCES

Frances had run a small store with her husband in the little town of Utica, Ohio. They changed homes but not communities. Frances knew the people in her town so well that she felt they were a part of her family. Between her many good deeds, hospitality and the veneration she gained by being one of the oldest members of the community, she was admired and helped by most of the residents. Her house ticked with antique clocks that my father-in-law made and every picture and piece of furniture held a memory of her husband, children, grandchildren and great grandchildren. She grew tomatoes in the same corner of her yard each year and stored food in her freezer for the winter. To pry her out of that house would have left her adrift. How would she ever get such support and love in a new community?

Her choice to stay in her home was reasonable. Her kitchen, bath, front room and bedroom were on the first floor. While she liked to go up and down the stairs to her basement to store or retrieve her canned goods or upstairs to occasionally clean or prepare for guests; she could handle the layout of the house. A little help with the furnace or plumbing was all she needed. She managed the lawn, gutters, and even painted her tin roof—amidst the protest of her three adult children.

If that's where your parent is coming from, let her enjoy her friends and home. Help her out wherever you can with your fix-it tools or whatever money you can spare to pay for a plumber and do keep in touch with weekly phone calls and regular visits. If you take her to a doctor appointment, it would also be a good time to talk to the doctor about her condition. She may be experiencing macular degeneration, crippling arthritis or memory loss that she doesn't want to discuss. Independent seniors often avoid telling their children of anything they feel may put them in a nursing home.

But a Frances parent is a rather easy-care parent. Just don't forget her as you tend to all the other people and duties in your life.

DONALD

If your parent is having serious health problems, such as chronic heart disease, diabetes or fighting cancer, then you have a very different situation from that of Frances.

As in the case of my father, you want to be sure that they are getting good health care. A single parent with health problems is going to need to look into nursing care in the home, residential homes, assisted living or a nursing home.

If their health problem is life-threatening, call a hospice group in your parent's community and see what they might advise.

On the other hand, if your ailing parent still has a healthy spouse who is willing to care for them in their home, as was the case of my dad, then he may be able to continue in his familiar surroundings with occasional visits from a nurse and, of course, you—his caregiver.

Keep in mind that my ailing senior father was married to my senior mother, so while she could clean up his messes, cook special foods, give him his medications, worry over the doctor reports and rub his back when he was hurting, Mom couldn't continue that for long without it taking its toll on her health.

And an added twist to their problem was that my mother couldn't drive. I had to make frequent trips to their house when my father's health was down so Mom could pick up some groceries and get to the doctors.

When we realized that Dad was going to continue to go in and out of hospitals and Mom would be his primary caregiver, my husband and I suggested that they sell the house they lived in for sixteen years and move into a retirement community that was closer to us. The retirement community had housing options that consisted of ranch homes with garages, apartments, assisted living and a nursing home on the same campus.

My folks had always considered moving to an *old age home*, as they put it, when they felt they might be a burden to my brother and me but they hadn't investigated any of today's retirement communities.

So one day I asked my parents to visit Copeland Oaks, in Sebring, Ohio. They liked the idea of renting a house on the campus with a garage and a sunroom off the back. The lawn would be mowed, snow would be shoveled and any home repairs or appliance problems would be solved by the retirement community. A bus could take Mom to the mall or grocery store if Dad wasn't feeling good or take them on a group trip to Lake Erie or Branson, Missouri—and there were lots of other amenities.

Copeland Oaks had a large lake stocked with fish, an indoor swimming pool and Jacuzzi, exercise room, free entertainment, library, an on-campus bank, beauty shop, woodworking shop, craft room, cafeteria, formal dining hall, an Acorn Shop for selling handmade items and a used clothing store with exceptional bargains.

Still, with all those wonderful services available to them, my 77 and 79 year old parents said, "I don't think we're quite ready to move yet."

One year later, when my father was going into the hospital about every three weeks and coming home with an oxygen tank hanging off his shoulder, they said, "Okay, we'll reconsider moving to Copeland Oaks but I don't think we can manage an entire house. We want to look at a two-bedroom apartment."

And so they did. The day we saw the apartment was the day my parents signed up for it. They were really happy. I guess it was time.

Fortunately, their house sold quickly and we were able to move them into their new apartment within about a month. Even though Dad was anxious about leaving his doctor, he was able to find a new doctor that got him off the oxygen tank. My father bought himself an adult tricycle and began to bike all over the campus and the town of Sebring.

Retirement communities are mushrooming up all over the country. Some have individual housing options and others don't, some are more expensive than others and some include the nursing home on the campus while others are located near a nursing home facility. Most of the retirement communities offer low-cost transportation, on-campus activities, emergency medical attention and no more yard or home maintenance.

So get on your internet: go to **Google.com** and look **up *retirement communities*** in the **state and city** you would like to have your parents move to. If you start gathering up information now, you might find the one that suits your parent's needs and financial status by the time they require it.

Don't let your parent tell you that they don't want to move into a retirement community with a bunch of old folks and nothing to do. Everyone we have talked to in the retirement communities we've visited have said they wished they had made the move sooner.

My husband and I have signed up with a retirement community nearest to our son. Even though we don't intend to move there for a few more years, it's nice to have our name on the list. We can always say no if we're not ready when they call us.

Here are some other advantages of a **retirement community**, especially if your parent goes there while they are still able to get around:

(1) If they go on a long vacation, their place is watched by friends and campus security.

(2) They are among lots of other seniors who are from the same era as they are, which means they share memories and careers that may not be what they are today. Eighty-year-olds may have worked on the railroad, been raised on a farm and danced to Glenn Miller's music. Likewise the seventy-year-olds on the campus will remember Viet Nam, President Kennedy and the rock and roll sounds of Chuck Berry and the era of Doo Op.

(3) Friendships begin quickly in these places because all the senior residents moved onto the campus in the last year or so. Remember what it was like when you first went to college or to a summer camp? Everyone felt a bit uncomfortable at first, and then you made friends with those who were once strangers to you.

(4) The friends your parents will make while they share activities like movie night, crafts, gardening, swimming, etc. become the community caregivers who take turns visiting your parent when they require a stay in a hospital, nursing home or during the grieving process after the loss of a loved one. It helps take some pressures off you when you have a large population of retired senior helpers.

(5) Also, these communities often have a "life care" provision to help assure the resident that they will still have a home, even if they run out of money due to illness or an unexpected financial set back.

(6) The generational "clashes" that often occur in a typical community are diminished if not removed altogether. No more boom boxes, late-night parties or cars racing down your street.

(7) Each residence in the community has an emergency contact feature (via a button or taking the phone off the receiver) to allow your parent instant medical attention.

(8) If one of your parents should wind up in the nursing home, the other aging parent doesn't have to drive through the rain or call their caregiver every time they want to visit their spouse, they just walk a few steps from their apartment to the nursing home or assisted living facility where their spouse is residing.

Like anything else, retirement communities need to be checked out. Since your parent will be signing on for the remainder of their life in this facility, you want to check out everything, including the nursing home portion of the campus.

Do understand that your parent does *not* own the house or condo in the retirement community. They are renting it. And there is an entrance fee on top of the monthly rent. The entrance fees may be rather steep, but a portion of it may be able to be retrieved if your parent moves or dies. So be sure to get all the financial facts clearly stated and discuss this decision with their financial advisor. *(Go to chapter 14 for our retirement community checklist.)*

The following pages will give you a glimpse into a few retirement communities in my state of Ohio. These are only a fraction of the retirement communities that you will find in my state or the entire country, but it gives you a preview of the fabulous options available to seniors today. And I would recommend that your parents look for a retirement community near their caregiver.

Copeland Oaks
800 S. 15th Street
Sebring, OH 44672
1-800-222-4640
www.copelandoaks.com

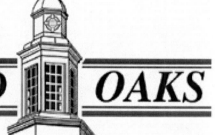

COPELAND OAKS

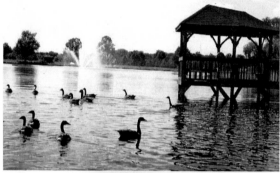

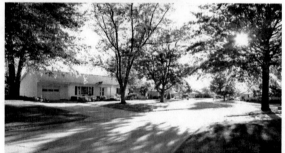

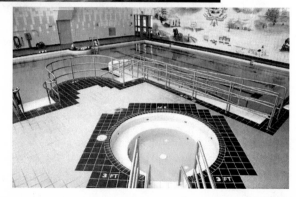

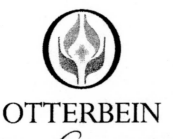

OTTERBEIN
RETIREMENT *Living* COMMUNITIES

Otterbein Retirement Communities
580 N. State Route 741
Lebanon, OH 45036
1-888-513-9131
www.Otterbein.org

Cridersville, Lebanon, North Shore, Portage Valley, and St. Marys, OHIO

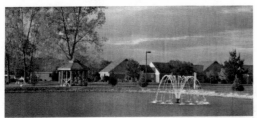

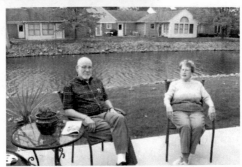

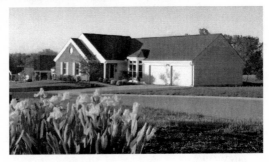

ALICE

And that brings us to the "Alice" portion of our housing issues.

Even though my Dad had some problems with his health, while they were in their apartment, Mom seemed to be able to take care of him. However, when the strain got too great I requested that my father be admitted to the nursing home on the campus for a short time where Mom could visit him and Dad could get the specialized care he needed. Then, when Mom regained her strength, Dad would come home and she would go back to caring for him.

After my father died, my mother turned their two-desk office into a craft room. She earned some money by sewing kitchen towels to hang over the oven door, treated her friends to her home-baked pies and enjoyed activities at Copeland Oaks as well as with our family.

Unfortunately, that only lasted about four years and my mother began to show symptoms of agitation and forgetfulness that was later diagnosed as Alzheimer's. Due to her poor eating habits and occasionally forgetting her medications, we were advised to consider the assisted living facility on the campus.

Unlike hospitals and nursing homes, patients have to volunteer to go to assisted living. To our amazement, Mom accepted the option and found herself enjoying assisted living more than any other place she had lived.

She had her prepared meals with other friends in the sunny dining room by the lake, her bed was made and her room cleaned every day, the nurse brought her medications on time and she was able to read more, color velvet pictures (which was her new hobby) and take walks around the well-landscaped grounds.

That lasted for almost a year, and then she began to roam.

When a patient begins to roam, they raise their risk factor for injury or exposure to the elements due to going outside without proper clothing or getting lost, so the doctor assigned Mom to the nursing home with an ankle monitor bracelet. As it turned out, she was amicable to that idea, even though it was emotional for us to see her thoughts deteriorating.

When we later moved to Columbus, Ohio, we also moved my mother to a nursing home facility closer to us. It worked out very well and she seemed more alert with our frequent visits.

While a nursing home may be the worst place you can imagine to put your parent, when the time is right, it often turns out to be the best situation for everyone. (*Review lists in chapter 14 and also you may wish to read the account of my mother's journey through Alzheimer's in my book,* **Inside Mom's Mind** *which you can find on my website, DonnaTrickett.com).*

Now, let's review your parent's housing options:

HOUSING OPTIONS:

(1) Your parent could stay in their own home:

- Good idea if your parent is physically and mentally in good health.
- If their home can accommodate their needs; has bedroom, bath and living space on the first floor, entrance to the house doesn't have many steps or the house is not too cluttered with furniture and things to make it hard to maneuver.
- Your parent is eating well, able to clean and remembers to take their medications.

If your parent needs some help:
- Healthy spouse, sibling, or adult child is willing and able to care for your parent out of your parent's home.
- Private caregivers from newspaper ads, the Area Agency on Aging and home care agencies are available. You may want to check out the National Association of Professional Geriatric Care Managers *(Be sure to check credentials, references, and conduct an interview and look at chapter 15.)*
- Adult Sitters *(mostly to provide companionship, do light housekeeping, make meals and be sure your parent gets their medications).* You may find them through personal references or a church bulletin board. Always interview someone you don't know and ask for a reference of their character and ability to care for a senior adult. Have them meet with your parent.
- MedicAlert® lifeline necklace. *(Note chapter 15)*
- Housekeeper *(to do light housekeeping, prepare meals and possibly run errands).* This may also be a "sitter" who stays all day or all night.
- Nursing assistant *(a certified nurse to give personal care; such as bathing, shots, dispense medicine, hook up any medical equipment, etc.)*
- Depending on how many things have to be done to keep your parent in their home; such as a ramp, a live-in care person, a visiting nurse and such, it may take an additional $500 to $1500 per month.

(2) Your parent could live in YOUR home:

- If your parent is physically and mentally in reasonable health.
- Great if you can have separate housing on your property for your parent, allowing you and them privacy and easy accessibility. (An adjoining room, a downstairs apartment that offers a same-level outdoor exit or a smaller home or trailer.)
- If you and your parent have a good relationship. That includes your spouse and children. Arguments could add to stress, divorce or senior abuse.
- Are you up to it or do you suffer back problems, insomnia, bipolar, diabetes, etc?
- Adult Day Care Centers (to watch senior adults who may have no one at home to check on them during the day). These centers can also allow you to run errands or just rest, knowing your parent is all right.
- If your parent's room and bathroom will be on first floor of your home.
- If your home does not have obstacles, like split levels, sharp-edged furniture or narrow halls.
- If there's not too much chaos (pets running through the house, teens blaring music or lots of visitors or people coming or going.)
- Does your job allow you time to take your parent to the doctor, talk and not neglect your other family members?
- Do you have the background (preferably nursing) to take care of medical issues?
- If they wake up and wander during the night, do you have monitoring devices in your home to know when they leave or where they are?
- Do you have to modify your home in any way; a ramp, special bathroom equipment and handles, etc?
- Is this decision going to cut you off from family members or friends, just when you need their support the most?
- Will it make a financial drain to your finances? Can other family members chip in to keep your parent part of the year or help financially?
- Cost-wise, you may be looking at an additional $500 to $1500 initially and then $200 per month expense by adding your parent to your household and of course that is not including any medical bills or necessary equipment which you hope to have covered by Medicare. (You should be able to use your parent's Social Security check and other

retirement income to help supplement your bills. Also, you would be able to claim them on your taxes if they were a resident in your home for the better part of a year. Check with their CPA)

(3) Your parent could move into a Retirement Community:

- Seniors are usually eligible to move into a retirement community at age sixty.
- Even if they don't feel ready today, you can get your parent on a waiting list and they can still say no if they are not ready to move when the facility becomes available.
- Retirement communities are open, active places that give your parent a variety of housing options and friends.
- Your parent should be able to keep their pet, their car and even a camper in the retirement community.
- Many communities have a "life care" plan (in case their money runs out) and an "out" plan (in case they decide to move to another facility later on).
- Try to locate your parents in a retirement community that is close enough to your home so that you can check on them and include them in your family's activities.
- These communities are great for all levels of care for the senior citizen.
- Retirement communities charge $1000 to $3000 a month and up, depending on what style and size living space they select. Houses cost more than condos. Condos cost more than apartments. And room and board apartments obviously cost more than apartments alone. But do remember this usually covers all maintenance costs to the living space, in and out; utility bills (except for phone or internet) and may include other addendums like swimming pools, transportation and free movie nights. Be sure to ask for details. Also, you don't have to pay property tax since you don't own the home.

(4) Your parent may benefit from an Assisted Living facility:

- Assisted living is great when a parent can no longer do all the necessary daily tasks (like bathing, dressing, eating or getting their medications on time.)
- The staff should include nursing assistants and registered nurses.

- Assisted living may cost $2000 to $4000 per month, not counting medical bills.

(5) Your parent may require a Nursing Home:

- A nursing home is necessary when your parent needs round-the-clock nursing care, even though your parent may be ambulatory.
- Nursing homes may cost from $4000 to $8000 a month, depending on the home, whether or not they have a private room and that does not include additional medical bills.

(6) Personal Care Homes or Residential Care:

- While an adult care person is always available to your parent in a residential facility, they may not be a licensed medical person. If your parent requires round-the-clock nursing care, this is NOT the facility for them.
- However, if they need help to be sure they get a hot meal, aren't alone and get all their meds when they are supposed to, this may be the perfect choice. It often has a homey atmosphere and is not as crowded as many assisted living facilities, so they will get more individual attention.
- Also, the cost is often very reasonable. You can expect to pay between $1500 and $3000 a month, and once again, that does not include additional medical bills.

(7) During the end-of-life issues, a hospice facility may be needed:

- In addition to hospice visiting your parent in the home or nursing home facility, hospice also has facilities for your parent to go to when it has been determined that they are near death.
- They receive round-the-clock care by skilled nurses offering your parent comfort to their body, mind and soul.

CHAPTER 10
Assisted Living and Nursing Homes

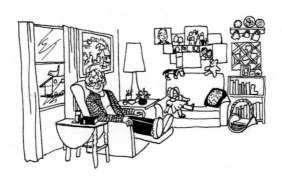

So you already have your parent in an assisted living or nursing home facility or you are feeling pressured to make that decision soon. Do you feel guilty about it? Is your parent accusing you of trying to get rid of him/her? Do people question your decision? Read **chapter 13, "Reducing the Guilt,"** to help you release yourself from that bondage. Also, **if you are dealing with a dementia or Alzheimer's parent, look over this chapter carefully as well as chapters 11 and 15.** They are chock full of unique ideas, from music to bird feeders, that can really make a difference in your parent's thought process.

Assuming you've had time to think about the matter of nursing homes and your parent's doctor agrees with you or has suggested the move, then let's look at how to make the one-room accommodation a more appealing place for your parent.

Let's have a Party:

Did you ever consider celebrating your parent's move into assisted living or a nursing home with a party at the facility? While that may sound strange, it was just the ticket for my senior Alzheimer's mother. It's a great way to introduce your parent to everyone and it makes your parent feel special. My mom got dressed up for the occasion and everyone came around to share in the festivity, including the staff. Let's look at what you might need to put together this "get-acquainted" party.

(1) **First get approval from the facility and set up a date.** It may not be the day your parent arrives but it should be soon after.

(2) **Look over the area where you are allowed to set up your party.** It may be the lobby, dining area or just a corner of a room at the facility. Decide how you will decorate and where you will lay out the refreshments.

(3) **Check with the staff about your planned menu.** Most facilities have no problem with occasional sugared treats but they may request some sugar free treats for their diabetics.

(4) **Plan your menu.** The facility may support your party by offering a cake or finger sandwiches. If not, consider a sheet cake with your parent's name on it and some sugar free cookies on the side. Ask the facility for some bottled water or hot water for tea or coffee and be willing to bring the tea bags. (By the way, you can get coffee in individual bags, too) Be sure to bring colorful paper plates, napkins, plastic ware, sugar, sugar substitute and packets of cream.

(5) **Plan your decorations.** Everyone enjoys helium balloons and your parent will be able to keep them in their room after the party to remind them of the occasion. Put up streamers and even consider cute favors, since seniors love to have keepsakes. Careful not to damage the walls or ceiling of the facility with tape or tacks and be sure any *favors* are safe for the senior residents. Soft mini toys and plastic window ornaments are often appreciated.

(6) **Consider having some old music to entertain the residents while they eat.** *(Suggestions in chapter 15)*

(7) **And if you feel so inclined, consider entertaining the residents with a sing-a-long or any other talent you or your children may be able to offer.**

Know what your parent likes:

(1) **What do they like to look at? What scenery, movie, flowers, birds or other favorite animal do they enjoy?** Besides pictures of family members, you can hang up large posters of their favorite subject. Most nursing homes allow pets to visit. Be sure to ask what conditions are stipulated in regards to pets (Updated shots, caged or leashed, friendly disposition, etc.). With a DVD player hooked up to their TV, you can have a couple of their favorite movies on hand to play at any time. *(Musicals, classics, travelogues of places they've been or wanted to see and DVDs of their grandchildren are great. Check out chapter 15.)*

(2) **What colors do they enjoy the most?** Consider getting them a new bedspread and door wreath in their favorite colors. Put up curtains and towels in their bathroom that goes with the color scheme of their room. Buy them a few outfits, pajamas and bathrobe in one of their favorite colors. And do consider how those colors will affect them.

Having studied art for over 50 years please let me add a word about specific colors and their effect on our emotions under my **COLOR POINTERS:**

- Bright **YELLOW** is the most offensive color because of the way it affects our eyes. Think of bright sunshine. While yellow is good for getting attention and can exude joy and energy while stimulating the intellect, bright shades of it should be used sparingly. Bright yellow paper is great to write on to leave a note for the nurse but it may create agitation in your parent if it is used to color the walls. Pale yellow or splashes of yellow in their clothing is a better choice.
- **RED** has always been associated with anger and romance for good reason. A bright shade of red actually increases the heart rate and blood pressure. Since seniors often have problems with their heart, use bright shades of red sparingly. Better to consider deeper shades, like brick red, which may exude a warm feeling, but even there, do not paint the walls with it. Soft **PINK**, on the other hand, which is a light shade of red is found to be very soothing and comforting. It has even been used in some prison settings to subdue inmates. So the shade of the color can make a big difference.
- **ORANGE** combines the energy of red with the joy of yellow. So combining the qualities of red and yellow will produce an equally

energetic powerful color that needs to be used sparingly. Once again, it is the shade of the color that can produce a host of reactions, from the depressing quality of dark orange to the elegance of gold.

- **PURPLE** has become more popular in the last ten years and lighter shades of purple (violet) have often been used in clothing for the senior adult. Associated with kings, purple combines the calming stability of blue with the energizing quality of red. Dark purple can be depressing, even frustrating, but violet (light purple) has a more reflective feminine quality to it.

- **BLUE** is also a calming color that seems to encourage thought. In other words, it may be a good color for the walls of a **dementia** patient who tends to feel agitated at times and forgetful. Too much blue, however, may be depressing. So mix blue with other colors in the room.

- Similarly, **GREEN** is a calm, reassuring, safe and relaxing color. It is referred to as the "feel good" color. But be careful what shade of green you pick and how profusely you use it. Yellow-green may take on some of the offensive traits of the color yellow while blue-green may serve to combine the calming qualities of both colors.

- **BLACK** can be good when used in small amounts for attention and power but should not be used as a piece of clothing near the face, it emphasizes too many flaws in an aging person. And never use black on the wall or on any large pieces like a bedspread or chair in a small room, since it can be depressing and make the room seem smaller. Since black is associated with death and mourning, it's probably a good color to avoid or at least use sparingly.

- **WHITE** is a powerful color exuding a sense of cleanliness, freshness and sterile conditions. While white can make a room look much larger, it needs to be mixed with warm colors that make the room more homey and welcoming.

- **GRAY**, **BEIGE** and **BROWN** are neutral colors and will go with most any other colors. There are many shades and hues of a gray and brown like blue-gray, gold-beige, chocolate brown, etc., so get a paint expert to help you if you are trying to decide on the appropriate wall colors. Gray is in the cool range of colors while the more masculine and stable color Brown depicts warmth.

- Darker colors tend to relax and may be depressing or allow brighter colors to stand out more (think of yellow dots on a navy blue background), while lighter shades of the same color may make a small room seem larger and brighter (such as sky blue walls), resulting in a more positive response from your parent, both mentally and physically.

(3) **Do they like visitors or do they prefer solitude?** If they like visitors, have a welcome sign on the door and some sugar-free treats in the room. If they don't like a lot of company, ask the staff if they can keep their door closed. *(Of course you do want to encourage your parent to participate in some of the activities at the facility; it keeps them more alert and sociable.)*

(4) **Are they into computers?** My father didn't care about the TV; he just wanted to type his life story on the computer. Today, many seniors would agree. While they may be in a nursing home, it doesn't mean they aren't able to handle a computer. So if your parent is computer-competent—work it out with the facility. Some nursing homes are even installing cable outlets for internet use. It can also keep them in touch with the grandchildren through their email.

(5) **Do they like birds or squirrels?** Bird feeders and even squirrel feeders are great additions outside the window of any nursing home room. You can get feeders that have a one-way mirror that juts into the room for an up-close bird show or one that attaches to the window and others that can hang from a tree or pole. Don't expect the staff to fill the feeder. And when you fill it, use only hulled sunflower seed since it does not leave a mess and it attracts a wide variety of birds. *(Note chapter 15 for resource places that handle feeders.)*

(6) **Do they like stuffed toys?** Believe it or not, aging women *and* men can find comfort in a stuffed toy. Many **Alzheimer's** patients think baby dolls are their children and others just enjoy the softness and warmth of the toy. I have seen men enjoy a life-sized toy dog and some patients just like to collect them as something to do and admire. Since they often exchange their toys or they may get them soiled, don't give them something that is too expensive or a keepsake.

(7) **Do they enjoy painting or crafts?** Most nursing home facilities have a craft or art day at least once a week. Art activities have been found beneficial to **Alzheimer's** patients because they seem to be happier and able to communicate through that media. You might want to attend one of the classes with your parent, if they are a bit reluctant to get involved.

Parents who might have once been quit social, may, with medications or mental difficulties like dementia, act shy or frightened and need a little nudge. Also, buying velvet pictures, which are attractive and easy to color with watercolor markers, may be a pleasant diversion between craft days.

(8) **Do they like music?** Have a CD player hooked up in their room that has headphone options, especially if they have a roommate or are hard of hearing. Then find their favorite music: hymns, old tunes from their era, show tunes, etc. Once again, music has been beneficial as a memory booster for **dementia** patients. The right music can also have benefits to their health. *(Note chapter 15)*

(9) **Do they play an instrument?** Many instruments may be too bulky for them to have in their room or handle anymore—like a piano, cello or drum set. However, most facilities have a piano in the dining hall or a lobby which they may be allowed to play. If their musical talent is really bad, you may want to encourage listening to music or finding easier to play instruments that are more manageable. Our 90-year-old friend enjoys playing in a kazoo choir. It might be something you could organize in your parent's facility. And, of course, always ask the facility for permission.

(10) **Do they like to exercise?** No problem. Most facilities have exercise classes and gardens for their residents to putter in or long hallways to walk in. (Check that your parent's facility offers these options since positive activities are important.)

(11) **Do they enjoy collecting things?** If the collectables are expensive, like rare figurines or coins, plan to bring the items once in a while for their enjoyment. But it would be risky to display them in the room. However, if the articles are stuffed toys, china cups or good books (not rare editions), find a display shelf for the wall or a narrow bookcase.

(12) **Does your parent like to work puzzles?** Don't frustrate your aging parent with anything too complicated. For dementia patients, you may want to consider a 50 or 100 piece puzzle or even a child's wooden puzzle. They are easy to handle and give instant gratification. And if your parent has painful arthritis, children's puzzles are easier to handle and some even have knobs to grab. Seniors like working on calm outdoor scenes or bygone days. Most

senior facilities have a table set up with a large selection of puzzles near by for the puzzle enthusiasts.

(13) What sports did they participate in? Display pictures of the sport or their achievements on the wall. If they liked a certain team, you can get them a bedspread or throw with the team's logo. You might want to add a sport-themed decoration to their door, like a wreath of golf balls, a tennis racket, or a toddler version baseball bat. It may take a little crafting on your part to get it to be a door decoration, but you will enjoy the results and they will appreciate your effort. *(Note chapter 11)*

Let's look at the room:

(1) DO THEY HAVE ONE OR MORE ROOMMATES?

This may limit the options you have for decorating and bringing privacy but you can improve your parent's living space with some cooperation.

(a) Ask the other roommates and the facility if your decorating ideas would be agreeable to them.

(b) Consider decorating the bedding, walls and window area to serve the entire room of patients.

(c) As to privacy issues, you may request at least a curtain divide be put up between the beds.

(d) And if your parent or another roommate is losing their hearing and turning up the radio or TV, consider providing headsets for each roommate.

(e) If nighttime gets noisy, with TV watching or snoring, consider a white noise machine which can override a lot of sounds. *(Note chapter 15)*

(2) ARE THEY IN A PRIVATE ROOM?

(a) If the establishment allows your parent to select the paint or wallpaper for the walls of their room, be sure to check over my **COLOR POINTERS** which was number 2 under the topic *Know what your parent likes* at the beginning of this chapter.

(b) Consider a cheerfully colored comforter or bedspread.

(c) Adding a small dresser and flat screen TV would save space. *(Remember, expensive items like a flat screen TV are not the responsibility of the facility. Since most bulky secured items in a nursing home or assisted living facility are not disturbed, it's not out of the question, but be especially careful with jewelry and cash.)*

(d) Note items you can make or buy in chapter 11.

(e) Hang a wreath on their door, to help them find their room and look welcoming.

(f) Hang pictures of family and other images they like on the walls.

(g) Put up a ribbon bulletin board *(chapter 11)* to display pictures and cards.

(h) Consider a leather or vinyl recliner chair that may even have a lift feature for easy sitting and exiting. *(Leather or vinyl is important because of the incontinence problem of seniors. Check out chapter 15.)*

(i) Hang stained glass images in the window, especially if they do not have a very good view.

(j) Put up a bird feeder outside their window to entertain your parent in any season. *(Feeders can attach to the window or hang from a pole or tree. Check out chapter 15.)*

(k) If they don't have room for a desk to write a letter or color a picture, consider a collapsible TV tray that can be stored next to their chair. There are also flat curved trays made to fit over the arms of the chair and then be set tight next to the wall. Also, most nursing home facilities have hospital trays in the room that can not only fit over the bed but be lowered to fit over the chair. *(Note chapter 15 for resources for trays.)*

(l) A small shelf with a railing around it mounted next to your parent's recliner chair is handy to hold small tissue packets, pencils, pens, crossword puzzle books, an eye glass case, sugar free throat lozenges and an address book in large lettering. *(Note chapter 15)*

(m) Do avoid having jewelry or other expensive items in the room or on their person. Small attractive items often get taken by the residents, and yes, occasionally by the workers. So consider purchasing faux jewelry if your parent insists on wearing their wedding band, expensive watch or other valuable items.

Keep your parent in touch with the family:

(1) If you live near your parent, even if they are retreating into Alzheimer's, plan to include them in family dinners and get-togethers. It will make a difference in everyone's life; you, your parent and any children who need

to observe how to care for seniors . . . because *you* may be the senior they care for in their future.

(2) To make it easier on your physically challenged parent, plan picnics at the facility's garden area or family dinners in the facility's private dining room.

(3) Make a DVD of your parent reading a children's book out loud and then send the book and DVD to the grandchild or great grandchild. It's also nice to include an appropriate doll or stuffed toy to go with the story. Video your parent holding the soft toy while they read. (Hallmark has also come up with a selection of recording books. Check them out at their store.)

(4) Put a series of digital family photos on a digital picture frame that will play over and over for your parent.

(5) Make mini albums of events that your parent participated in or would have liked to attend, but couldn't. Label each album with what it is about (Mike's Wedding, Our Trip to the Zoo . . .). Label the pictures of the people in the album with the names of each person right on the picture, along with their age. If your parent attended the event, be sure they are in some of the pictures. Leave the album with your parent to enjoy. (*It really helps dementia patients to feel that they aren't forgotten, even if they can't remember the event.*)

(6) Ask the great grandchildren to send their crayon drawings to your parent.

(7) Encourage letters, cards and postcards with enclosed pictures to be sent out from all the family members. Ask them to print or type the letters in large print so your parent can read them easily.

(8) Letters that are meaningful or express gratitude for the sacrifices and help your parent gave to a family member is really a thoughtful way to communicate love to someone who doesn't feel useful anymore. (*These letters are also comforting to the family members to read about their parent after they die.*)

(9) As your parent's caregiver, be sure to send out pictures and brief summaries of your parent's condition, so they have a reason to write back. You might

even include a self addressed stamped envelope with your personal letter to insure that your parent gets a response. Emailing has become a substitute for letters and cards, but since your parent won't be receiving emails, these letters are precious. Also, include any inquiry your parent may have had about the person. Ex: "I hope John got that job he wanted", or "How is Mary doing in college?" It will put a personal twist on the letter that most people will respond to.

(10) Ask visitors NOT to bring live plants or cut flowers. They will get spilled or not get watered and they can breed mildew. The best flowers are silk. They look great and you don't have to worry about them.

(11) Have small packages of your parent's memorabilia gift wrapped and waiting to be given to a visiting adult child, grandchild or great grandchild. Your Mom can tell the children about the significance of the object and the family member will feel special receiving these items.

(12) Have little toys in your parent's room for any visits from small children (great grandchildren or visiting church friends). Put the toys back in a drawer for the next visit.

(13) Have other toys gift wrapped for small children who don't visit often, (like great grandchildren) to give to them to take home. It makes a visit to a nursing home more enjoyable and memorable.

(14) Be sure your parent has treats in colorful tins to give to children or other guests. Ex: Flavored jelly beans, mixed individually wrapped sugar-free candies. *(Sugar-free is a good idea since your parent will probably be nibbling some throughout the day, even when there isn't any company. It gives them a treat that shouldn't hurt their diet.)*

(15) When children visit, have a small blanket to put down on the floor and some sanitary wipes to clean them up after the visit.

How to help get better care for your parent:

To help your parent get more attention from the nursing home staff, be sure to leave some treats at the nurses' station or in your parent's room. (A tin of cookies, a box of candies, a couple pizzas, a container of specialty coffee or some homemade goodies can brighten the eight-hour shifts of these exhausted professional caregivers.) Remember to include some diabetic treats for those who require them and don't forget the night shift, they are often the busiest of all. Also, little gifts to the nurses during short hospital stays can bring more attention to your parent, which is especially helpful if your parent suffers from dementia or Alzheimer's.

Create a Nursing Home Outreach for ALL Ages:

An outreach project (which is a pleasurable activity that brings comfort and joy to the residents) can make those routine weekly visits a bit more pleasant for you and your parent as well as your family. And you don't have to put on a show every time you visit . . . just once a month or once every other month.

While an outreach activity is done for the entire facility, you may want to include your parent in your show or at least arrange for them to be in the front row. All outreach activities need to be approved by the facility as to the date, time of day and what you plan to do, before barging in. So call ahead.

We have found that right after lunch is a good time, before they take their afternoon naps. If you go room to room, don't stay more than 15 minutes. And if you are doing this for a group of residents, often in their dining hall, keep the activity between 30-60 minutes. Ask how many you can expect to attend. We have found it averages around 30 patients.

There are great outreach projects going on in your local churches. If you don't have a clue where to begin getting one started for your parent's assisted living or nursing home facility, you might want to join one that already exists.

Some outreaches to nursing homes do formal Bible studies. We haven't found that to be very effective because the senior residents are often not alert enough to follow conversations or readings. Other more positive outreach projects have been to come in and play an instrument, read or tell a story or just pass out refreshments while you chat with the patients. (You must be sure any refreshments are approved of by the facility since diabetes or allergies to caffeine or chocolate could present a problem).

The most effective outreaches my husband and I created included **music, laughter, children and hands-on experiences.** Let me give you a brief sampling of some of our outreach projects so that you may confidently venture out on your own.

IMPORTANT

Especially when you add children to your mix, have some kind of **sterile hand wipes** for you and your cast to use BEFORE you enter the nursing home, *so you don't spread colds and such to the residents,* and for AFTER you leave, *so you don't take any germs home with you.*

And **do NOT let any persons go into the nursing home if they are just getting over the flu, are sneezing, or think their child may have or is just getting over a childhood disease**. Simple childhood diseases can be very serious to the elderly.

(1) SING-A-LONGS and RAFFLES:

You can do this one alone or with a group of any-aged persons. Just come in with a CD player, some old time music or hymns and some soft cute things you may have or you found on discount (that's for an optional raffle). Have the facility set up the people in a given area where you want to sing, and presto, you have an outreach.

I like to get acquainted by opening with a raffle. Just make up as many as 50 cards with large numbers on them. (Most gatherings at nursing homes are about 25-40 people, but ask the staff how many you might expect. I prefer making my own raffle tickets because the long small numbers on the commercially sold raffle tickets are hard for the seniors to read.) Be sure you have a duplicate copy of the number you pass out to put in your "hat" to draw the winning number from.

I usually go around my house and gather up about five or so little items that might cheer up a senior resident. Plastic window hangings and mini stuffed toys go over well. Open this outreach by handing out raffle tickets and asking patients their name and what they did for a living or how many grandchildren they have. (Don't ask "How are you?" This could lead down a depressing long list of ailments that would put a damper on your objective.) This gives you something to do while you may be waiting for the nurses to wheel in the last patients. Wrapping the gifts also adds to the excitement.

Pick music that the residents would know. Since most of the patients are probably in their 70s, 80s and up, look to the 1940s and hymns for your musical selections. Don't get too melancholy and be careful the song isn't too risqué. Amazingly, there were some PG-13 tunes back then.

(2) CLOWNING:

Create a character; it doesn't even have to be a clown. Colorful wigs help get attention and dressing like characters out of the past will wake the audience up. Try imitating Charlie Chaplin and the Keystone Cops or you may want to dress in an old fashioned outfit with a large lacy hat and gloves. While getting into a colorful costume might seem unimportant, we found that seniors get more excited and listen better when they perceive you are special. Just a fun hat or colorful jacket will work too.

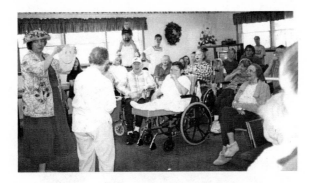

Once you are comfortable with the character you have created, find some fun stickers to place on the residents when you introduce yourself to them. (**Be sure to stick the stickers on clothing—not their skin.** We found seniors often can not produce the normal oils in their skin and it can make it hard to remove the stickers.) Have a kazoo with you to hum along with a tune and some music to sing to the residents that can be a hymn like, "Give Me That Old Time Religion," or a silly tune like, "She'll Be Coming Around the Mountain." Anything they are familiar with and can sing along with you.

Some silly illusions and puppets are fun and entertaining, especially when you can get the audience involved. If you clown alone, a **puppet** can be a good companion to talk to and respond to the audience. Check costume shops for the **"red velvet bag"** and the **"duck pan"** illusion. The owner of the store will show you how to do the illusions which will definitely get the attention of the audience. And there are lots of places to get puppets of every size and description. Check out the internet. Illusions and puppets are also great to get kids involved in the show. *(Check out chapter 15)*

Don't be surprised if a patient asks you to pray for them or you may want to ask if you could pray for them. Surprisingly, many seniors see clowns as entertainers from churches (which is often the case, since there is a trend today toward Clown Ministries.) By the way, if you do decide on a "clown" costume, don't be surprised if a few of the residents reject you. We have found that some people have "bad" memories of encounters with clowns while others beam with the excitement of a child.

Whatever way you choose to clown, be a "gentle" clown in a nursing home setting. Not loud or obnoxious. We would approach the door of a room and knock gently, wave timidly and ask politely, "Would you like a visit from Grandpa Buttons?" (Or whatever you choose to call yourself).

(3) YOUTH TALENT SHOW:

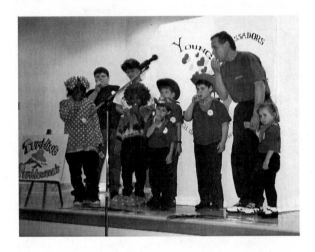

You can organize this group of young people through your church, neighborhood, your child's scout troop or just the children in your own family. My husband and I made up a family youth outreach that encouraged the parents of the children to participate. We worked together with a mixed group of children, five to eighteen, and adults up to 65.

Some did the backstage work of keeping the young ones quiet in a lobby area and lining up the performers to come in when announced. Others helped get the costumes on or pass out the props and still others, usually the teenage boys, worked the microphone, became the master of ceremonies, handled the CD player and any lighting effects. (By the way, **don't use a strobe light**; the flashes of light have been known to interfere with a heart pacemaker.) Interestingly, many of the teenagers we worked with were inner-city kids and half of our crew were teen guys, so I know this can be done.

One of the "hooks" to get the teens involved is to include **technical stuff**. Like I just mentioned, ask them to "gently" watch after the little ones and encourage them, let them create some skits for the program, show them how to use awesome **puppets** like Axtel® Puppet Creations and the integration of some believable **illusions.** Oh, yes, **teen boys like to wear beards, mustaches and sideburns.** They make great Charlie Chaplins and the Keystone Cops.

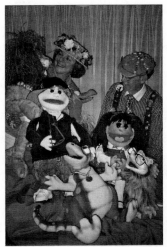 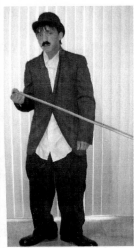

The **teen girls loved to wear wigs and glittery costumes** and they made great Andrew Sisters who can mime to the recordings. *(Check out chapter 15)* And they loved working with the children.

The **young children** loved the attention but they had to follow instructions and cooperate and be quiet as they waited to perform or they wouldn't be in our next performance.

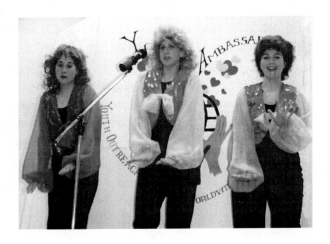

The way we put together a talent show was to have anyone who wanted to perform in the show submit an index card with their name, the name of their act, and the name of the tune they would play or sing. If they needed a CD to accompany them, they had to submit that to us with the card.

We had pre-rehearsed opening and closing numbers (which were group sing-a-longs) and some mini-skits that told a joke or did an illusion between the acts. Everyone was encouraged afterwards to pass out stickers and say "hi" to the residents. After several shows, we found the kids felt comfortable enough to carry on conversations with the residents and even push wheelchair patients back to their rooms.

Another thing that made these youth outreaches enjoyable was to stop and eat together after the show. Sometimes it was to go to Pizza Hut and other times it was to have an ice-cream cone at the Dairy Queen. Some people even donated money to the outreach to pay for props or meals out. You may not eat out every time, but set up this perk at least once in a while.

By the way, you can also get more people involved in this project if you ask for volunteers to make note cards or sock dolls to pass out to the residents at the end of the show (a pair of socks can make two dolls). Don't know how to make a sock doll? Just go to **Google.com** and type in "sock doll."

Obviously, a production like this can only be done once a month or less. If you did it more than that you would probably lose a lot of your participants and you might feel a bit burned out yourself. But I have to tell you that when we did this youth outreach once a month and the weather or our health prevented us from keeping an engagement, the teens would pester me as to when we were going out again. They really liked it.

The benefits of doing outreaches are astounding. Your parent will be proud of you, the children and participants will experience the joy of serving someone else and they may even make a new friend in the group that they didn't know before. (We discovered one of our Caucasian teen boys helping a five-year-old African American girl to learn her part.) The kids gained confidence, because you can't find a more appreciative audience than seniors in a nursing home, the children learned compassion for the elderly and the seniors often put smiles on the children's faces with words like, "God bless you, sweetheart" or "Aren't you a lovely child." It taught all the age groups to cooperate and appreciate each other.

CHAPTER 11

Stuff to Make or Buy

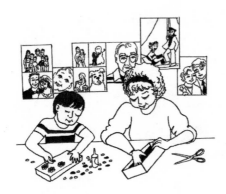

This is the fun chapter. You can go shopping or do handmade or computer-made crafts that can be done with family members, friends, young children and yes, even your teenager. And all of these things will help your parent while giving you a bit of a break from your official duties.

TIPS for GOOD HEALTH

Medical ID Cards that fit in a wallet.

Make a set of all three cards on the next page for your parent and fill out the medical forms in chapter 14 to give to the doctor, hospital and the facility your parent is residing in. Enlarge the cards on the following page to 160%. Each card should be 4" X 3 ¼", which will fold over to 2" X 3 ¼".

Medical ID Cards

These three Medical ID Cards should help speed your parent through the emergency room at the hospital, and give an EMS worker a quick *heads up* as to immediate treatment in the ambulance.

After you complete these cards, make two sets, one for yourself and one for your parent to carry in their wallet.

DIRECTIONS

(1) Make a copy of this page. You may want to copy each card on a different colored paper. (2) Carefully fill in the blanks by hand printing with a black pen, or use typewriter, or create these cards on your computer and update them as any medications or addresses change. (Use 8 pt. Times New Roman for title fonts and 12 pt. Arial Narrow for the information fonts.) (3) Cut out the card, fold and laminate it or cover it with clear Contact paper.

Emergency Medical Card

Name	Issue Date
Address	DOB:
	Hm. Phone
Primary Insurance & number	Living Will?
Secondary Insurance	
In Emergency call:	DNR?

Medical Alerts:

Medications:

Allergies:

Medical Problems:

Doctor or Doctors & Phone numbers:

Medical Alerts are: implants, anticoagulants, etc.
Allergies are: to drugs, pollens, bees, foods, etc.
Medical Problems are: heart condition, hypertension, etc.

Medical History Card

Name:		Issue Date:	
Surgery, Accident, Illness..	DATE		Town & State

Family Medical History Card

Name	Issue Date

Mother:

Grandmother on Mother's Side:

Grandfather on Mother's Side

Father:

Grandmother on Father's Side:

Grandfather on Father's Side:

Brothers and/or Sisters:

HOSPITAL SUITCASE

This should be a small carryon luggage that can be pre-packed and placed in the closet of your parent's residence. Let the head nurse know that it is in the closet and it's best if it is a bright color with an ID tag that says: **Hospital Suitcase for:** [and then print your parent's name and place of residency and YOUR name and title (daughter and POA) and YOUR phone number]. If your parent should ever need to be rushed to the hospital before you are able to arrive, the nurse can give the *Hospital Suitcase* to the ambulance workers.

IMPORTANT

LABEL EVERYTHING
with your parent's name & YOUR phone number
(YOUR phone number should be more reliable than your parent's.)

Items to pack in the suitcase (Keep paperwork* updated):

(1)   **A copy of POA papers* over your parent's health.**

(2)   **A copy of DNR papers*.**

(3)   **A copy of the Living Will*.**

(4)   **A copy of all the vital statistics* found in chapter 14.**

(5)   **Toothbrush** or denture brush and **Toothpaste** or denture cleaner.

(6)   **Containers** for dentures, glasses and hearing aids, if necessary.

(7)   **Hair brush and comb.**

(8)   **Deodorant.**

(9)   **Mirror** that can stand up by itself on the hospital tray.

(10) **Simple makeup.** *(Avoid nail polish because of the strong odors and doctors look at nail and lip color to check for health problems.)*

(11) **¾ length bathrobe.** (Full length robes may cause them to trip.)

(12) **Slippers** that they can easily slip into when getting out of bed.

(13) Cozy, attractive **night gown or pajamas.** *(Hospitals prefer night gowns that open up the back. Check chapter 15.)*

(14) **Picture of loved one** to put on night stand. *(Be sure the picture is a copy and the frame does not contain glass.)*

(15) A **prewritten card or letter from you.**

(16) Their favorite **magazine, crossword puzzle, Bible** or other religious material *(which is especially comforting when in the hospital. Be sure to look for the largest printed material available.)*

(17) **Writing material** so they can write a letter or note to someone.

(18) **Extra pair of glasses** for reading or distance, depending on their needs. *(If they aren't reading but will be in bed watching TV—you might consider distance-only glasses to help them see the TV better.)*

The RIGHT CANE or WALKER

If your parent needs a cane or walker, you'll find there are quite a few to choose from, so have your parent use the item in the store before buying it. Look for canes and walkers in a drugstore chain, Wal-Mart, a medical supply store and there are various catalogs that sell a variety of models. *(Note chapter 15)*

REMEMBER, most medical equipment purchases ordered by a doctor will be fully reimbursed by Medicare but do ask the supplier first, since the more elaborate versions of walkers or canes may not be covered.

Be sure to put their name and YOUR phone number on the cane in case your parent leaves it in a restaurant or store. It happens.

If they only have trouble with their knee or hip occasionally, they may want a light sturdy adjustable aluminum cane and it wouldn't hurt to have a collapsible cane that can fit in a purse, under the car seat or in a shopping bag for when their legs give out in the middle of an outing.

Besides the standard cane, there is the quad-cane with 4 legs at the base; while these are more stable, they can be a little awkward to manipulate.

The standard walker is collapsible and can fit in any trunk. It helps if they have sled-like skids or tennis ball covers on the back so your parent doesn't have to pick it up each time they take a step. But have your parent go for a test run, because wheels or skids can slip out from a shaky patient's stride. The high-end walker models, with flip-down seats, hand-brakes and baskets are usually not covered by Medicare and they may be confusing to an Alzheimer's patient. Test them out.

The RIGHT PILLOW

An aging parent often has trouble sleeping and doesn't always know why. Sometimes it's poor circulation in the legs, too many daytime naps and sometimes it's arthritic pains in the joints.

An extra pillow tucked between their knees and between their arms when they lay on their side may help. Be sure it's a soft pillow that has some form to it. I prefer foam but some may have trouble with the content, others think they create too much heat. Remember, the skin of an aging patient is thin and sensitive and often will bruise easily; so try to empathize as you patiently allow your parent to test various pillows out for the right softness.

Also, your parent may prefer a body pillow or a contour pillow for the head so they can breathe easily and get proper head support. There are soft, medium and firm pillows filled with polyester, down feathers, Styrofoam beads, foam, memory foam, and organic buckwheat. There are even pillows with built in speakers so you can listen to music while you sleep and others that have cool packs to keep you from overheating. With the right pillow, your parent may be able to get a better night's sleep and that will improve their health and mental condition—and you may discover the right pillow for yourself. *(Check out chapter 15)*

The RIGHT MATTRESS

Another obvious elephant in the bedroom is the mattress. Many individuals wonder why they have backaches and never consider that it might be that 25-year-old spring mattress that sags and squeaks every time they roll over.

There are so many new and improved mattresses today to choose from. You just have to take your parent into a mattress store and try them out. In fact, you may want to try out your parent's bed before embarking on the mattress hunt, just to know what they have been dealing with.

Also, even though senior couples don't like to be separated after sharing the same bed for forty or fifty years, it may be one of the reasons they can't get a decent night's sleep. If one partner snores, overheats or has physical problems, getting separate beds or even having them sleep in separate rooms might resolve their problem and make them less grumpy in the morning. Even a temporary separation when one has a bad cold may benefit both of them. If they are anxious that they may not hear the other if they have a need, consider baby monitors or night stand intercom for ease of communication.

Help your parents to realize that it doesn't reflect on their love for each other, only their need for a good night's sleep.

EYEGLASSES

Your parent probably has bifocals. Did you consider this? Often an aging parent will misplace their glasses or spend hours in a recliner chair or hospital bed, unable to see the TV through the close-up lower lens of the bifocal.

Solution: Buy several pairs of reading glasses from the drug store so you have replacements when one pair becomes lost or damaged. Have one pair near their chair, another next to their bed and still another in their hospital luggage. Buy several pairs of *distance-only* glasses for watching TV, which will have to be made by an optometrist. Their eyes should be checked every two years since the aging process can alter their vision more rapidly than a younger person.

Memory Boosters

If your parent is having trouble remembering, don't try to play the teacher and keep repeating names or dates in the hope of helping them remember, it can be frustrating for both of you and be of little value to their retention skills. However, these memory boosters may help:

SHOEBOX MAILBOX

To help your parent remember to keep all their bills, important mail and even items they would like you to order for them in one place—make a gaudy *shoebox mailbox*. Your kids or grandkids will enjoy this one. If your parent is in assisted living or a nursing home, they may not receive any bills or important mail but it's still good to have this box for anything they want to show you (a card from the grandchildren or a magazine clipping).

(1) Cover a shoebox with durable paper or cloth, since it will be used over and over again.
(2) Using tacky glue or hot glue, attach plastic jewels, silk flowers, or any items that appeal to your parent and will get noticed.
(3) Ask them to put the box in a prominent place and remind them to put ALL mail and magazine clippings in the box so you can find their bills or order something for them.

MEDICATIONS

One of the problems with aging, even without dementia, is forgetting what day it is or if you took your medications on time. Often seniors have more than one medication and it needs to be taken at a specific time of the day. Here are two helps that I found with my parent's and my own medications:

(1) Since it saves money to buy medications in bulk (often a 90 day supply), take the medications out of the bottle and put them in an air tight zip lock bag. (Be sure to push the air out before sealing, it keeps the pills from breaking down in the moist air. But keep the bottle for future pharmacy refills.)

(2) Purchase a pillbox that designates the day of the week and the time of the day that your parent needs to take their medication. You can fill the pillbox when you visit and your parent only needs to look at the open lid to know if they took their meds on time. *(You may want to have a calendar for them to check off next to the pill box. Pill boxes are shown in the catalogs I've noted in chapter 15.)*

TAKE LOTS of PICTURES

Pictures with the names, dates, and ages of the individuals on or under the picture are wonderful keepsakes, a gentle memory boost and lots of fun to put together. And the best pictures will show your parent in the scene surrounded by their family. *(Hint: concentrate more on close-ups of the face and facial expressions rather than the entire scene.)*

The following suggestions are ways to incorporate those pictures into your parent's environment and therefore their memory:

DIGITAL PICTURE FRAMES

You can put an entire album of pictures into these frames and your parent will enjoy sitting back and watching the images of his/her loved ones slowly change from frame to frame.

MINI PICTURE ALBUMS

Fill lots of small albums with pictures of outings or family activities that your parent will want to review again and again.

Label the album with the name of the event or activity. (Staff members at the facility find pictures a way to open conversations.)

RIBBON BULLETIN BOARD

These can be purchased from most retail stores that carry household goods or craft stores. They are great for displaying cards and photos because they don't need tacks or magnets which might get lost or stuck in your parent's foot. If you want to customize one to fit a narrow or very large space, you can make one out of plywood, polyester fill, fabric, ribbon and upholstery tacks. Just study the commercial designs and have fun with your creativity.

Put cards, pictures and children's drawings up on the board. Since most seniors do not get a lot of mail and may be suffering from some form of dementia, rotate the images periodically to make it seem like they have new items. Also, include printed names on the front of any pictures or inside the cards, so they know who it came from. You may have to also identify them as "Your son" or "Your grandchild."

FOAM BOARD PICTURE POSTER

(1) Purchase a 30" X 40" piece of *thick* foam board, available at arts and crafts stores. Thicker foam warps less.

(2) Copy and enlarge original pictures of family members to 5" X 7" or 8" X 10"

(3) Glue pictures to the foam board with acid-free glue sticks in an attractive arrangement.

(4) If you want to cut the foam board around some of the pictures to make a more interesting shape, not just one big rectangle, use an electric breadknife. Also, you may want to cut out a section to custom-fit the wall space, allowing for a wall switch or thermostat. (Craft stores also sell heated wire devices to cut through foam)

(5) Attach a button to both ends of a 2 ½ foot mounting wire.

(6) Use duct tape to adhere the wire to the back of the picture. (The buttons will help prevent the wire from slipping through the duct tape.)

(7) Hang foam board grouping on the wall with only one nail.

(8) You can add other pieces of foam pictures on top or off to the side of the arrangement as new children are born or grandchildren marry.

BUY SHELVING

While that may seem obvious to most people, sometimes the duties of a caregiver blind us to the practical solutions.

Since space is precious, especially in assisted living and nursing homes, going *up* by utilizing bookshelves is a great way to display your parent's memorabilia, collectables, picture albums and books. Screwing them to the wall can prevent accidents, but ask the facility first.

Look around; there are step shelves, long shelves, plate-holder shelves, cup-holder shelves, spoon-holder shelves, thimble-holder shelves and even glass encased shelves to reduce the dust factor.

There are also fold-down desks that have glassed-in display shelves above them with dresser drawers below (secretary desk). Bookshelves can be narrow enough to fit into a one-foot space or be a part of a night stand or lamp stand. *(Check out chapter 15)*

MUSIC & OLD RADIO SHOWS

Music is soothing and can help an Alzheimer's patient relax and recall things they may have forgotten. The right kind of music can also lower blood pressure and heart rate.

Locate music from your parent's era or musical taste: (Bing Crosby, Mozart, Hymns . . .). And consider old radio shows of Amos and Andy, Jack Benny and George Burns and Gracie Allen, because there is undeniable therapy in humor.

If you look through some catalogs and stores, you will find a record player that looks like an old fashioned radio. Many of them even play CDs and audio tapes. What a great way to play the old tunes and let them listen to their old records, if they still have them. *(Check out chapter 15)*

OLD MOVIES & DVD HOME MOVIES

Get your parent a DVD player. If they are not able to operate it, most staff people can. Buy old movies, not necessarily black and white but movies like *The Sound of Music* or *Meet Me in Saint Louie*; those were my mother's favorites. Old movies can restore the memories of the way life used to be, resurrect an old actor in the prime of his life, old tunes that remind your parent of a more pleasant time or just the enjoyment of a non-violent innocent movie.

And if the family can send DVDs of the grandchildren, great grandchildren, weddings or family get-togethers . . . especially with your parent in them, they will cherish them and remember. You may even want to use these as a personal touch at the inevitable funeral.

DOOR WREATHS

Door wreaths are not only inviting but they help a dementia patient identify their room. If it doesn't confuse them, you may also wish to change the wreaths with the seasons. You can buy commercial wreaths in a variety of themes and designs, from brilliant floral to wood-carved welcome plaques.

For a more personal touch, customize a door wreath to your parent's interest. Here are some ideas:

(1) Buy a grape vine, foam or straw base wreath from most craft stores.
(2) Wrap it with a garland or hot glue leaves or flowers onto it.
(3) Then, depending on the hobby or interest that your parent enjoyed, hot glue objects that reflect them. (Ex: golf balls, paint brushes, flower pots, knitting needles, etc.)

EASY DOES IT

COMFORTABLE CHAIR

Since your parent may only have room for ONE chair, you want to make it just right for them. Consider the following features:

(1) Most nursing homes will only accept vinyl or leather chairs, due to incontinence issues. For removable washable cloth recliner chair covers that add warmth, *check out chapter 15.*
(2) A recliner is good for getting their legs up but be sure it works easily, since an aging parent's arms aren't as strong as they used to be. *(Some electrically operated chairs have push buttons to raise and lower the legs.)*
(3) If your parent is having trouble getting in and out of their chair, you can get a lift chair at a medical supply store and it may be covered, in part or whole, by Medicare.

(4) Some chairs also offer heat and vibration. (If your parent has some form of dementia, you may not want to complicate the use of the chair with too many options.)

(5) Be sure you measure the space it will have to fit into before purchasing it. Also, recliners that can be placed right up against the wall (zero clearance wall huggers) help conserve space.

(6) Be sure you have measured your parent's leg length to the knee and knee to the floor, as well as their torso. Best if your parent can actually try it out before purchasing it because each recliner is made differently. Some are made for tall people, while others are made for short or even wide individuals. *(Check out chapter 15)*

COLLAPSIBLE TV TRAY

Have a collapsible TV tray next to the chair. It will allow your parent to have a writing desk or eating area that can be put away easily. The glider-style tray seen on TV and most stores is great because it can easily be pushed away from the chair and it has a lip to catch any spills. Of course, if they are in a nursing home or assisted living facility, they will have a large hospital tray on wheels. You can also purchase flat trays that rest on the arms of the chair and can slip tight against the wall when not in use. *(Note chapter 15)*

MINI SHELF NEXT TO CHAIR

If your parent is in a rather confined area, this small shelf, with side rails all around, will hold mini tissue packets, eye glasses, pens, colored markers, TV Guide, crossword puzzle book, etc. It's better than an end table because the contents won't fall off and it doesn't take up much space in the room. *(Note chapter 15)*

NIGHT LIGHT

If your parent should wake up disoriented or is in a new surrounding, a night light is comforting and practical. While you can get some really nice-looking night lights, you may also want to consider some figurines that use fiber optics to bathe the object in a soothing display of changing color. My mother really appreciated a fiber optic angel.

SPECIALTY PHONES

Your parent will appreciate a phone with large buttons and an amplifying receiver, if they can't hear well. Some of these specialty phones have a place for a picture of you or someone else on the button your parent may need to push, in order to speed dial the person.

Jitterbug® phones are great if your parent is still independent and finds the regular cell phone hard to work (because of small buttons) or general confusion when operating them. Jitterbug® phones also have a live assistant at the other end to help your parent use the phone. Who knew there were still real people who answered phones.

There are also emergency dialup phones and devices to get quick help when your parent needs it. *(Note chapter 15)*

CHAPTER 12

Spiritual Issues: Finding Peace

(Discuss the following information with a clergyman.)

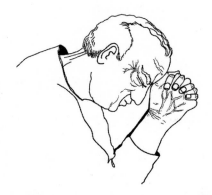

If there's one issue that gets stronger with age, it's the spiritual part of your life. Many seniors start going to church again or begin attending for the first time. Some begin serving the community and God in missions of mercy. Many feel they have come to understand the reason for the tragedies in their life. They feel closer to God and His thought process. They are at peace with life, even if they are experiencing heart failure, an amputated leg, and/or they are lying in a bed in a nursing home. I know because my husband and I have often frequented nursing homes and we have met many contented and spiritually inspired people there. I guess it's because they're getting older and death seems more eminent and less threatening, so they genuinely seek their Creator and a life after death.

TRUE STORY

My mother had to leave her three-bedroom home with a sunroom off her large kitchen and a dining room filled with her prized dishes and furniture in order to accommodate my father's health issues.

After my father died, Mom drifted into Alzheimer's and had to reduce her living quarters once again to a large one-room assisted living apartment with an adjoining bathroom.

As her disease progressed and she required nursing home care, she had to give up even more of her possessions to fit into a very small room with a very small bathroom. Her belongings were reduced to one chair, a bed, a dresser and a TV. Yet, when we came to visit her, soon after she was assigned to her nursing home room, she said, "This is very lovely. Everyone's been so nice to me. And I really don't need any more than this."

MORAL: Is your parent content and thankful? Then they probably have their spiritual life in pretty good order.

However, if you find your parent in overall good physical and mental health and not taking a drug that may cause depression and they're still despondent—suggest that they speak to their clergyman.

If they aren't attending a place of worship, you might introduce them to *your* clergyman or a friend of theirs who is a pastor. You may also want to have them talk to a counselor who is sincere about spiritual matters of the heart. I'm not talking about finding a sanctimonious person who likes to sound religious, I'm talking about a caring, compassionate believer who may be able to identify the source of their problem and help them find peace.

It may be that your parent feels guilty for something that happened a long time ago and they're afraid they aren't forgiven. It's often easier to talk to a stranger than to family about private matters.Maybe your parent never thought about something that happened years ago, until now. And since the person who offended them or they offended may be dead or no longer around, they feel an anxiety inside that won't go away. Sometimes they need to say a last goodbye to someone or they may just want to see a loved one for the last time.

My mother clung to life for eight days, to the amazement of the hospice workers, because she hadn't seen my brother during her final days of struggle. Bill lived in another state and though he had visited her earlier and talked to her on the phone, she missed seeing him.

We weren't sure that was the case, since my mother had Alzheimer's and often forgot our names or our visits, but at this particular moment in her ninety-first year, she was too weak to speak. The idea that she was waiting to see Bill was based on the suggestion made by the hospice nurse, who said, "Is there anyone that your mother may not have seen recently that would be causing her to hang on so desperately?"

My brother came immediately and hours after his visit she died peacefully.

TRUE STORY

My father had been an elder in our church for over 20 years. He read his Bible every day and you didn't want to disturb him when he was in a moment of prayer, which could be anywhere he was quiet with his arms folded and his body turned toward a window. While his temperament and language weren't always sterling examples, Dad was dedicated to being honest and responsible.

At the age of 80, when only ten percent of his heart was functioning, he begged us to pray for him. He was always strong and able to quote scripture. He even conducted a Bible study group. But this was different. He knew he was going to die and there was something that haunted him from his past. I don't know what it was—but it was there.

Dad pulled his weakened body down from his bed and knelt on the cold linoleum floor. Still attached to his IV, he prayed for God to forgive him and let him die. Then he got up and asked me, his youngest child, "Do you think God can forgive me?" I assured him that He not only could—but that He did. Nevertheless, I could tell in Dad's eyes that he was still not sure.

MORAL: No matter how spiritual your parent may be, they can still have doubts. I don't think you have to worry about their spiritual destination because they have those doubts. Wait until *you* have to face death. End-of-life issues are the expertise of most clergymen, so if the doubt is still lingering after your reassurances, bring back the pastor for another private visit and prayer.

Nelson's mother went through months of infections, heart failure and even two amputations at the age of ninety-one. It was hard to imagine how she could endure so many major invasions to her frail body but she kept on fighting until she heard that her granddaughter had given birth to a healthy little girl. She had grown very close to this grandchild and wanted to know the final outcome of her pregnancy. Frances died within days of hearing that everything had gone well.

Our spirit is an amazingly powerful force that needs to be nourished.

Many of us, at one time or another, may have doubted that there is a heaven or that God loves us but when you're over 80, either your faith gets stronger or the doubts get even bigger. Your parent may be looking for reassurance and not just some kind words but solid belief and scriptures to back them.

If you don't think *you* can handle that job or because you're battling some hurt that your parent did to you years ago and it's clouding your compassion, it's time to seek the experts.

MDs, unfortunately, usually don't have the time to get to the bottom of such issues and will probably prescribe a tranquilizer or sedative for your parent. General psychologists may only look at the clinical side of their depression and also prescribe some medications. However, Christian psychologists or clergymen can often discover if there is a spiritual hurt that needs to be addressed. They may still recommend a doctor but they may give you more insight into the cause of your parent's unexplainable depression.

And don't forget the help we got from hospice in the area of care as well as spiritual advice. If you've tried to cheer up your parent with a family outing, their favorite food or a delightful old movie that you watched together and they still remained despondent, it may be any number of medical conditions—or it may be a spiritual need. Don't overlook that possibility.

CHAPTER 13
Reducing the GUILT
(Use the following information to forgive yourself.)

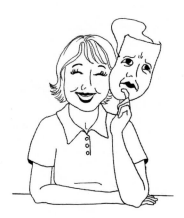

Nothing can be more debilitating than guilt. It ruins your sleep and leaves you powerless to accomplish anything. In short, guilt can drain the joy out of you. And when you lose your joy, you lose the greatest gift you can give your aging parent and yourself. Mom can get her medications from the nurse, her hair styled by the beautician and her checkbook balanced by an accountant—but your hugs and positive conversations are priceless.

If you're feeling guilty for not visiting enough, not being as devoted as your sibling, for past arguments you may have had with your parent or for being too busy on that fast track we call *midlife crisis*, you may need some help to shake off those shackles of condemnation. Guilt could even put your life out of balance as you place your aging parent at the head of all the other individuals and responsibilities in your life.

While there will be times when your parent should take center stage due to an emergency or other real need, you have to balance your time. A little time for your parent; a hunk of time for your spouse, children, grandchildren and friends who will become your support system during and after your parent's death; time to help others outside your family and necessary time for yourself to revitalize your mind and body. Also, I have found that I must be sure God is in my daily life or I become overwhelmed and depressed.

Guilt destroys but forgiveness restores. And that forgiveness has to start with forgiving yourself and then forgiving anyone who has laid some heavy guilt on you. Then there is the forgiveness you may have to give out to an abusive parent in order to feel free inside. After you gain your mental peace, you can serve your parent better and not worry about what others expect of you. So let's look at some of the guilt that may be burdening you:

Compared to other caregivers, I feel that I don't visit my parent as much as I think I should.

Now where did you find a timetable that designated the amount of hours you're supposed to spend with your parent?

Maybe your sister visits your mom everyday and you *feel* that you should do the same. You may have watched a reality show that had an invalid parent living in the home of their child and it made you *feel* terrible that your parent is in a retirement facility. A senior friend of your Mom may make her *feel* that kids today don't care about their aging parents. Notice all of the above comments contain the word "feel" and feelings can be deceptive. What you or your parent feels may not be reality.

Truth is that today's official caregivers do a lot of work behind the scenes. You may make important phone calls, shop for needed equipment or personal items, move your parent to a new home or facility, balance their checkbook, mow their lawn or look after their dog while they're in the hospital. Does your sister or neighbor call the doctor every time there's a question about your mother's medications or pick up the adult diapers on sale at Walmart? Probably not. Some designated caregivers live in another state and are only able to see their parent once every few months. Whether you have your parent living in your home, visit them in a facility every day, once a week or every three months—there is no right or wrong caregiving schedule.

Of course we do need to be aware of that old deceiver, *Procrastination*. It's so easy to make excuses in order to not spend time with an aging dementia parent. After all, they may not know your name or remember you visited the day before. Maybe you don't like nursing homes, watching your parent's health and mind decline or the fact that your parent is no longer able to communicate well. No one does.

After a challenging day with my Alzheimer's mother or enduring a round of angry outbursts from my aging father, my husband and I found it refreshing to stop at a restaurant to talk and eat on the way home. I don't recommend eating out every time you visit your parent, it could increase your waistline or reduce your wallet, but you need to find a trusted friend with whom you can unwind, shed some tears or even blow off some steam.

You have to work out your caregiving timetable according to your other personal obligations; your health, financial situation and the difficulty of having to watch your parent's decline. No one knows what you feel like inside but you. Just do *your* best and don't worry about the actions or opinions of others.

But what if I did NOT have a good relationship with my parent and now I am their caregiver?

That's a tough one. I had that dilemma with my father. He was not a cuddly kind of dad. Though he was an honest, faithful and brilliant man, he could often hurt with his words. While his angry outbursts were usually followed by an apology, the pain of his words was branded in my heart.

After my husband's retirement and the empty-nest stage of my life began, my father appointed me POA over their money and health. When Dad's physical condition declined dramatically and his temper still flared up, I had to wrestle with the past hurts and the distasteful duty of listening to his continual criticisms that were hurled primarily at my Mom. For hours after our visits, I unloaded my pent-up frustrations on my husband and found myself in constant silent mini-prayers to God in order to help me prioritize and stay focused.

Years later, when Dad was assigned to a nursing home, I found him sitting in a wheelchair by the nurses' station in an adult diaper as his gaunt cheeks collapsed while sucking a chocolate milkshake through a straw. My compassion poured out to him. Without my Dad asking forgiveness for his past and present behavior, I forgave him.

I continued to help my father as I became his ambassador, creating peace agreements with the nurses who were complaining about his conduct. I found that having candy roses in a vase next to his bed was a great way to thank the frustrated nurses for their undying service to him. Dad discovered you could get more attention with sweets than with rage and I was making regular shopping trips to the candy store.

Amazingly, in the midst of all this, my father and I began to heal years of hurt. It took fifty-four years, but it felt good to be able to hear my father say *thank you* and hand out compliments and even smile more. For that reason alone I was glad I had the opportunity to serve as his caregiver. I hope you will find a similar conclusion to your service as caregiver to your difficult parent.

Despite the not-so-good memories you may still harbor, take a deep breath, say a quiet prayer and forgive your parent's past actions. As hard as guilt is to bear—sometimes forgiveness is even harder to give. As I said earlier, *forgiveness*, requested or not, is the real answer to your frustration. The benefits are enormous. Forgiveness will stimulate an inner peace that destroys pent up anger and could lead to your own health benefits.

I feel guilty for not wanting to visit my parents because of all the stress I feel when I leave their home.

As I said earlier, I understand. Often I would go to my parent's home to help in some way only to watch them get into a squabble over some trivial matter. Dad would often be irritated with something my mother did or didn't do, she'd defend herself in tears and then it would escalate. If I jumped in to help mom, as I did so many times when I was a child, I only intensified the fight and then I would leave in defeat. Let's face it, not all parents act like June and Ward Cleaver from the *Leave It to Beaver* series.

Ideally, you might want to suggest a therapist or marriage counselor for your parents but after fifty years of repeating their destructive behavior, do you really think things are going to change?

My mother had been in that kind of relationship for nearly sixty years and she never asked for help. She often called me to complain but she would not come to our home for even one day to let Dad cool off, nor would she let anyone else care for him, except when he was hospitalized. While my mother's commitment was commendable, her willingness to accept unfavorable conditions was not.

Needless to say, things can get rather distasteful when you are looking after an aging parent who is losing control of his life. When Dad felt powerless, he would lash out over the tiniest things. Once he got mad at a glass of milk he knocked over, shouting that it was top-heavy and poorly made, leaving Mom to clean up the mess.

If you have to walk into that kind of tension each time you visit or if you are expected to endure heavy smoking, drinking or even illegal drug use while you are with them, you may *have* to reduce your personal contact with your parents in order to serve them.

As to what to do for your parent when their behavior gets really dangerous, such as driving while intoxicated, taking illegal drugs or causing your mother physical injury, you're going to need a good domestic violence counselor. Even though you may have heard that seniors mellow with age, and they often do, sometimes due to changes in medications, escalation of personality issues due to fear and mental problems of the aged, some parents can become more violent. A serious case of parental abuse toward their spouse and caregiver is recorded in the book, *Elder Rage (look at chapter 15 for details)*. While my father was not that bad, he did make my job as caregiver a bit more challenging.

If it's at all possible, I do encourage you to not *stop* your visits all together. You may have to stop them for awhile because you may have become the catalyst that escalates a disagreement but eventually try to come back for a visit because, catalyst or not, your parent loves you. Even when they say, "Get out of here!" they don't mean for good, they only mean that they want you to not add to their problem by taking sides.

You may not be able to go on a vacation with them like you've heard your friends do, spend an overnight at their home or even an entire day together. Instead, look for a helpful neighbor or service group, such as a visiting nurse or adult daycare that can make sure your parent has a safe place to go and that they get their medications. With outside help you may be able to find enjoyable moments to share together—or not.

Since fewer visits from you will probably create more friction with your parents, describe why you need to reduce your visits. It may help to explain that you love them both and it upsets you to watch them bickering all the time, so you've decided to reduce your visits and get other duties done for them out of your home.

If you feel you can deal with them better in a public setting than in their home, periodic outings to a restaurant, shopping, a park, etc. may be your answer.

Just like a child, you may have to warn them in advance about fighting in public and that you will be reducing their *playtime* with you if they do. I know that sounds like you are the parent and they are the child but it sometimes turns into that scenario when your parent grows older and may be experiencing their own unique set of problems, from dementia to arthritis.

While one of your parents may have endured the stress of an abusive relationship, you do not have to. Be sympathetic but firm.

My mother feels I'm not doing enough for her. She constantly compares me to her neighbor's adult child.

As I mentioned before, I don't know of any timetable or duty roster that tells you what a caregiver should be doing. In the case of my mother-in-law, she was able to be very independent and chose to live alone after her husband died.

She paid her bills, made it to many of her doctor appointments by herself and managed the house and yard, even after turning ninety.

Her one son, who lived closer to her, would visit once or twice a week. We managed to get there about once every two months but my husband did chat with her on the phone every week. Her daughter, who lived several states away and was having health problems, was able to visit her mother once or twice a year for two or three weeks. Who was the better caregiver? All of us. We did the best we could within our circumstances. How did each member of the family perceive the caregiving qualities of the other? I don't know and it really doesn't matter.

Parents, especially mothers, who usually have stronger emotional ties to their children and grandchildren, will often play the *guilt card*. You know the one. "The neighbors have asked why you don't come to visit more." "I hope you're coming soon because I baked your favorite pie and Mother's Day is just around the corner." "Son, could you help me paint the house?" "Your brother changed the oil in my car yesterday (hint, hint)."

Think of those comments as words of love. I mean, after all, she just wants to visit with you. She misses you. In the midst of those guilt-inducing comments are the words, *I love you.*

And don't underestimate Dad's love for you. He may be quieter about the emotional portion of his life but aging often makes a man turn to mush. Just watch him with the grandkids. The truth is that he would like to see you and the kids more often, too.

Before you think I'm laying more guilt on you, all I'm saying is don't get upset if your parent lets you know they care about you in some awkward way that may make you feel they're scolding you. They may even shout at you and say, as my mother did one day when she phoned me and had to leave a message on my answering machine, "If that's the way you want to act towards your mother . . . not answering your phone . . . well, well, I disown you!! You're no longer my daughter!!"

Did she really mean that? Of course not. True, the words stung a bit but if I got insulted to the point of not calling her back, where would that leave me now, five years after her death?

Thankfully, I was able to get past her words. I called to explain that I loved her but I couldn't always be ready to answer every call or be there the minute she wanted me. I promised her that I would visit the following week and then Nelson and I popped some popcorn and watched an enjoyable movie together—with no guilt attached. And yes, I did visit the following week. We went out to dinner and did some shopping. It was a good day.

I'm not a real happy person, especially when it comes to seeing my father in a nursing home, so how can I be a cheerful caregiver for him?

Well, I'm sure your parent already knows who you are, personality wise and otherwise. After all, they raised you and we can't all be sanguine (upbeat personalities). So don't worry about the cheery part but you can still think of things to do with or for your parent that can make their day a little more pleasant.

Consider a trip to the zoo with the grandchildren, a visit to the conservatory to see beautiful flowers in the middle of winter, share a meal with them at their residence or change their environment by going to a restaurant. Even slurping an ice cream cone together on a hot summer's day can make a big difference for both of you.

Avoid talking about your shaky job or the terrible economic conditions in the world. Instead, remind them of the fun you had together on a trip to the beach when you were a child. (Try to find some old pictures and bring them with you when you visit.) Your parent will enjoy knowing that they helped to plant some good memories in your mind and heart and you'll be surprised at how much it will help you to think more positively about your own life.

Visit on a day when the activities director is doing a craft that you can participate in. You can also ask the facility if you could come to entertain the patients. If you play guitar, can teach a craft, have a knack for telling stories, want to bring in a friendly pet which has all their shots, bring along a talented child who would like to sing or play the piano or you want to lead everyone in a sing-a-long to some old tunes on a CD player, most nursing homes welcome those interruptions. Also, I have found that my parent was more involved when I was the one leading the activity. *(Note outreach ideas in chapter 10)*

These are also good ways to get your children and grandchildren engaged in their aging grandma's life. Before you know it, you, the somber one, are making an entire facility smile—even if it's not your normal persona.

I know I'm not as good a caregiver as my neighbor. She has her mother living in her home.

Good for your neighbor. Maybe they had a close relationship throughout their lives together and having her mother living in her home is like sharing with her best friend. Maybe her mother is in good health and able to help around the house. Perhaps economically it is the only feasible solution for her and her mother or maybe your neighbor is feeling guilty for their past relationship and believes she has no choice but to bring her mother into her home.

Whatever the reasons your neighbor is choosing to have her mother live in her home really doesn't pertain to you. The very fact that you accepted the duty of caregiver and that you're reading my book to better serve your parent is evidence that you're doing a good job.

You never liked being compared to other children in school or in your family, so don't compare yourself to other caregivers now. Do the best *you* can. All you can expect of yourself is *your* best and the best you can be is much better when the guilt factor is removed—or at least reduced.

My mother has a lot of health problems and needs professional help. She says if I really love her I will never put her in a nursing home or a retirement community.

First of all, your mom will be assigned to a nursing home by a doctor if her health gets to that stage. You really don't have a lot to say about it. Yes, at one point your mom may be able to be cared for by a visiting nurse, out of your home, but please read on so that you take into consideration all the issues involved in that decision.

One real consideration if your parent is not seriously ill may be found in chapter 9—the **retirement community**. Your parent will have lots of activities, friends, walking paths, therapy classes, immediate medical attention, as well as transportation for trips and other outside events. Frankly, we plan to move to a retirement community in the near future.

After my grandfather died, my grandmother decided she wanted to live with one of her sons. That meant she had to leave the retirement community they had lived in together, filled with daily activities and friends, and move into our home. She thought it would keep her close to the more active beehive of her children.

Truth is our home was isolated at the top of a hill with no stores or walking paths. Her arthritic body needed help to get up and down the stairs. Since my parents were at the *empty nest* stage of their marriage, they just wanted to enjoy some quiet time together. My grandma would get restless and create problems as she felt lonely without her friends or activities. Due to her loss of bladder control and her refusal to wear diapers, she created messes for my mother. What was going to be a bonding time for my grandmother was turning into an endurance test for everyone concerned.

The Waltons TV series created a cozy family scene that we would all like to replicate. We joyfully watched this large family work, eat, sleep and play together during the tragic period in our nation's history, the Great Depression.

The grandparents, Zeb and Esther, shared in the work and teaching of the six children. They talked, cried, hugged, and were aware of each other's daily joy and tears. It made you want to say, "Why can't we live like that today?"

First of all, while the Waltons program was created out of some true life experiences of the author Earl Hammer, it was in fact fiction. And it was from a time that doesn't exist today in America. Drugs and gangs were rarely an issue. Biological family members lived under the same roof, which is almost nonexistent today. Grandpa was able to help with the family business, which was right on the property, so they didn't need an extra car to get to work. Grandma was a capable and willing cook, housekeeper and instructor for the children, plus Zeb and Esther gave their home, business and land to their family to live on because it was given to them.

There was no mortgage to pay off and because the Waltons lived on a farm and grew their own food, their grocery bill was minimal. There were no malls or credit cards to go in debt to; no cell phones to interrupt every hour of their day and their entertainment consisted of one radio that everyone gathered around in the evening. Does that sound good to you? Perhaps so, but does it sound like your present home and lifestyle?

Here are some factors to consider before agreeing to move your mother into your home: How safe is your home? How mentally or physically challenged is your mother? Does *your* job or health allow you to give the care your parent will need when the nurse isn't there? (*Carefully read over the issues in chapters 9 and 14.*)

Another very important point that you need to consider is your family's dynamics. After all, we're talking about an aging parent with health problems entering your home—not a puppy. Caring for seniors is draining enough to any eldercare nurse but it's especially taxing for a family member. And your parent may play that *guilt* or *sympathy card* more effectively with you than they would with a professional nurse.

If you know that having your parent live in your home will create a rift between your spouse and your children, then it may be a bad idea. It could lead to a divorce or even senior abuse.

A Christian friend of ours, who had an abusive father, decided it was time to bring his aging dad into his home and mend some broken bridges. Our friend spent a bundle remodeling a room in their home just for his father. It had a fireplace and an adjoining bathroom. Our friend's wife cooked delicious meals for her father-in-law but he never seemed to appreciate them. Their young daughter was constantly being criticized by her grandfather until she cried. After several months, they could no longer endure his behavior and they set him up in a retirement community. It worked well for everyone.

Let your mom know you love her, that you'll visit her regularly and you'll take her places. Assure her that she won't be left alone and that you will do everything you can to make her place comfortable and her experiences pleasant. Then be sure to back up your words.

Like many children going to their first day of kindergarten, Mom may cry and even say things that hurt. Nevertheless, if you keep your promises and she begins to settle into her new surroundings, she will eventually thank you—or not.

My father had an aorta transplant when he was 68 years old and triple-by-pass surgery at 70. We tried to convince my parents to move to a retirement community where they wouldn't have to worry about clearing their icy steps in the winter or mowing their lawn. They both insisted that they were too young and so they went back on the road in their camper. At 78, my father was having difficulty breathing and endured several more surgeries. Finally, they consented reluctantly to the idea of moving to a retirement community.

Two weeks after they moved in, my father said, "Thank you. This was the best thing that ever happened to us." He actually got better and was out riding around on an adult tricycle.

When my mother required the assisted living area due to her Alzheimer's progression, she was anxious and fearful. She felt she would lose her friends and have nothing to do. Within minutes of arriving in her newly decorated room, my mother beamed with contentment because it lifted so many burdens from her mind. She no longer worried about taking her medications or what she would eat—that was all done for her. She took walks, read books, visited friends, did crafts and went on trips. She was content.

Look over chapters 10 and 11 to get some ideas about how to make a nursing home situation a bit more enjoyable and chapter 9 for housing options.

Even if Mom doesn't thank you, you know you've done the best you can. That's all you can do. Really.

Mom says that whenever I talk to her about end-of-life stuff, like wills and POAs, she feels old and that she's going to die soon.

My mother-in-law was 84 years old when we brought up the issue of having all her paperwork in order. My father had just died and I was thankful that he and I had done all those necessary things to insure that my mother would be able to live out her life with as little hassle as possible.

Nelson's mom sounded favorable to the idea of having her oldest daughter, who was her POA, go over any suggestions we had made. I put together a quick list of about eight things that I felt were important and said that Loretta could call me to discuss anything she might not be aware of. His mom said, "Fine, I'll have her do that. Thank you."

The next thing we knew we discovered an angry phone message on our answering machine from Nelson's brother that said, "You've really upset mom. She's crying and saying that you made her feel like she's going to die. What did you say to her?"

It took a few hours on the phone to get the whole matter straightened out but it all boiled down to a fear that my mother-in-law had about getting old.

According to the guidelines for AARP membership with regards to age, if you're over 50, you're a senior citizen. And since as long as we're alive we know we will eventually die, it really doesn't matter what age we are, death is our inevitable end. But then, you knew that and this isn't about the reality of her situation, it's about her perception.

A good place to start helping your mom with her end-of-life issues is to take care of your own end-of-life issues and then show her the paperwork. Explain how much more freedom you have and how peaceful you feel about your future knowing that you have lined up all your financial, legal and medical ducks.

Another good time to bring up these issues is after the funeral of a family member or one of their friends. After seeing how someone else's funeral was conducted, you may be able to open up conversations about funeral planning and such with your parent.

If that doesn't work, call other family members in to help get those issues settled. Hopefully your parent already has their will, POA papers, living will, etc. in order. But if anything mentioned in chapter two is not complete, it may be time to finish the job with the support of your family.

Old wills, insurance policies and other legal papers may need to be reviewed in regards to beneficiaries and whomever they may now want to appoint as executor.

Then if that still doesn't move your parent to complete these important tasks, you'll just have to get the ball rolling anyway. Set up an appointment with an estate lawyer and let him know of her reluctance. Ask him to be encouraging and even flattering if need be.

Once your mom gets to his office, she probably won't complain in front of the lawyer. And after the lawyer compliments her for being a wise parent for taking care of all that legal stuff, she may change her mood quickly—or not. Again, you have to get past her feelings and realize that these papers are essential to giving her the best care and ensuring her wishes are carried out.

Dad has been driving since he was 16. I know his eyesight and responses aren't what they should be but I hate to take away his last vestige of independence.

Would you rather see your dad in a hospital or on trial for having injured someone after a car accident? I know this is a very touchy subject and your dad is possibly furious about your even suggesting that he should give up his car—but safety is paramount.

While your parent may not be aware that a certain medication's side effects could negatively impact his driving, are they aware of just how serious that could be to them or another driver or pedestrian on the road? How would your dad feel if he knew he injured or killed another person because of his negligence?

My mother didn't drive but my father did. After backing up his car, full speed, into another car and jamming it into the wall of a store, his insurance went skyrocketing and our concern was on high alert. I told Dad that it was time to think of giving up the car keys but he insisted that it was only his new medications which were causing the trouble and that he would be okay once his body adjusted to them.

A few weeks later he made another bad judgment call by running into the bumper of the car in front of him and we had another talk. On my request, Dad took both the driving and written test again, and to my amazement—he passed. However, as his heart began to get weaker, he realized that driving with an oxygen tank off his shoulder wasn't the best idea. We convinced him to move into a retirement community, where my non-driving mother and he could catch a bus or hitch a ride with a friend when they needed a lift.

So what should *you* do? Basically, pay attention to the signs (such as an accident or traveling 40 mph in a 65 mph zone) that tell you it may be time to relinquish the car. Then sympathize but be firm with what needs to be done next. Either elect to have them retested (written and driving) or get the doctor to state that they should not be driving due to an illness such as epilepsy, impaired reaction time, visual problems or mental instability. The raised insurance rate along with the added cost of owning and maintaining a car may also help to convince them to give it up.

You must understand that they will feel stranded and alone without a car, so you need to assure them that you will find ways to get them to the doctor, the store, their friend's home or even on a little trip now and then. Either you need to provide this service, along with the help of your other siblings, or provide them a residence where vans, buses or car pools can get them to where they want to go.

If *you* had to give up *your* car, what would you do? I guess caregiving comes down to the golden rule we learned as kids. *Do unto others as you would want them to do unto you.* Hey, it works.

My parent is having health problems and my spouse wants to take a vacation. I feel guilty to have fun when Mom's not well.

I know how you feel. There were lots of times that my husband and I felt guilty for going to a movie or taking a trip when one of our parents weren't feeling well. After over ten years of caregiving for both my parents and helping my husband's parents, we can say that you just have to do it.

First of all, be sure that your parent is getting good care and has access to emergency help if needed, either in a senior residence, MedicAlert® button or a hospital. A simple cold when you are 85 may turn into pneumonia, so you need to be concerned about their physical complaints.

Sometimes your parent may not actually be sick, they just want some attention. It may be that your visits are too sporadic, and if so, try to cut out some time from your busy schedule on a regular basis to drop in on your folks. Even put it on the calendar. Take your parent out to dinner or over to your house for a get-together. Visit them as often as you can and be sure their health needs are being cared for (via a visiting nurse or facility) but don't deny yourself or your family a chance to relax and have fun.

After rather simple laser surgery to my eye one morning, I asked my husband if we could drop by the nursing home to spend a little time with my mother. I thought it was only going to be for about an hour. Unfortunately, on that particular afternoon, my mother had a recurring bout of her bleeding ulcer and our short visit turned into a hospital ordeal. I was tired, angry, even a bit irritated that my mother's problems were invading my life.

I mentioned to one of the interns that I needed to rest after my surgery and he said, "You can leave any time you want, Miss, we'll take care of your mom." Those words cut into my heart. Here I was complaining about wanting to get some rest when my mother was in severe pain and confusion. I stopped complaining and stood by her until 2 a.m. when she was finally assigned a hospital room. She was going to have more tests run in the morning. After a restless night's sleep, I felt ashamed and thought I needed to give more of myself to the care of my mother. But there wasn't much more I had left to give.

In truth, I was at the end of my proverbial rope that day. I needed a break. I had stayed with Mom and fought the medical system to see to it that she had good care. While my feelings were understandable, I needed to allow myself some time off.

We are human. We get tired. Caring for an elderly senior is draining but caring for a sick elderly parent can lead to emotional burn out. Just when your parent needs your smile and encouragement the most, you may be exhausted and filled with tears. So grant yourself that vacation or even a quiet dinner and movie night together with the other loved ones in your life, who will be there after your parent passes on. Don't take the guilt with you on your outing. Dump it.

I can just about guarantee that when you visit again, after the fun time with your spouse or family, you will be able to enjoy your parent more and give them a refreshing smile instead of a miserable beaten down look of defeat.

Since my Dad had a stroke, I make sure I never go anywhere without activating the call—forwarding feature on my cell phone. Even though I'm exhausted, I feel guilty if I'm not available when the nurse calls.

Unless you are working with hospice and you know your parent is in what I call "the dying place," where they could pass away at any moment, you really are taxing your adrenalin and nerves to be on-call, 24-7.

What if you did get a call that your Dad had another stroke or even died unexpectedly—what would you be able to do about it? Are you an emergency responder? Did you know that hospitals and ambulance crews take the doctor or crew member off the case when they learn that they're related to the patient in some way? It's because, even someone trained in how to respond to a medical emergency can get caught up in their emotions and not perform as well.

Emergency teams and nurses in nursing homes don't work around the clock. They work in shifts, often getting more than one day off at a time. They need to get rested, eat a few good meals, get some exercise and even have a little fun. It gets them ready for the next emergency.

If you find that you're gaining weight from turning to those wonderful comfort foods we call junk food—or losing weight because you can't sleep, eat or you're just running too much—you need to stop and think. If you continue to push yourself to be on call, 24-7, where are you going to wind up? Probably a hospital or at the very least, feeling irritable and tired. And how is that going to serve your Dad if he needs a new doctor or a new treatment? How clear will you be thinking to make those decisions and how cheery will your next visit be?

You taking care of *you* is as important as your Dad getting his meds everyday. Remember our first point? Your hugs and positive conversations are important gifts to your parent. When you take care of yourself it actually FREES you to be a better caregiver. Lets take that word **FREES** and substitute a word for each of its letters.

F = **Fun**
R = **Rest**
E = **Eat right**
E = **Exercise**
S = **Sleep**

Yes, you actually need **FUN** in your life in order to feel joy in your heart and mind which prompts you to do enjoyable things with your parent. So go have fun.

REST is not like sleep. REST is that quiet feeling that allows you to recline in your favorite recliner chair without feeling your foot twitch because it's anxious to be doing something. REST is that guilt-free baby-like nap in the middle of the afternoon that allows the phone to be unplugged while you stretch out and close your eyes with a smile on your face because you've allowed the pressures to be put on hold for an hour. Oh, okay, you can leave the answering machine on but you don't have to respond to it.

To **EAT** right doesn't mean to eat healthy foods while you're on the run, nor does it mean to eat junk foods while you're sitting in a quiet restaurant. You need healthy foods, in right portions, as well as water (not coffee or pop) in a quiet setting with, preferably, good company. I know that's a hard one and I'm still working on it myself, but you know eating right helps your thinking, health and appearance.

And **EXERCISE** is also important to your mood, your health and your appearance. It's another toughie, especially when your own knees hurt or you're running around in the car all the time. Try walking around the block or use the stairs and not the elevator. Exercise with a friend. Talking while you're walking can be great for your marriage and it helps to straighten out your thoughts while accomplishing your exercising goals. I find that biking on my adult tricycle causes less stress to my knees.

Finally, remember to get enough **SLEEP**.

My pilot husband could get up at 4 a.m., drive two hours to get to work, sleep in a hotel room on a lumpy mattress, leave a distant city on the last leg of his trip at 8 p.m. and get home at midnight. At 6 a.m. the next morning he bounded out of bed with lots to do around the house and never seemed to weary. That was when he was in his thirties. Now, at seventy, he gets 8 to 9 hours of sleep and sometimes takes a nap in the afternoon. It keeps him healthy and happy. That's important to both of us.

If you're getting only 5 to 6 hours of sleep at night, you're probably saying, "It's all I need," but is it? Are you feeling anxious? Did you come down with a cold or flu last winter? Are you taking sleeping pills or other medications for your nerves? Are you finding that the only way you can get up in the morning or stay awake all day is because of that cup of coffee? Are you forgetting things? You may be worried that you have Alzheimer's but chances are it's because you have too much on your calendar—or is it your Blackberry?

This high-tech information age has children text-messaging on their cell phones while surfing the web on their computer. We feel that everything is important and we can't let one piece of information get past us. Truth is, some of it will get past you (and it should) and you can't be everywhere (so don't even try).

Just because your parent is getting old and they are experiencing senior issues doesn't constitute a twenty-four hour alert. Keep up your regular visits, talk on the phone, check with the head nurse occasionally, but don't become obsessed by your parent's problems. A doctor or hospice worker will alert you to the really life-threatening issues and then you may have to be more vigilant.

It's good that you take your caregiving duties seriously but don't sacrifice your health and family. Your parent needs you, your family needs you and a lot of other people you call friends need you. So be sure there's something left of you when the drama of caregiving is over.

I got DNR-cc (do not resuscitate-comfort care only) papers for my mom and now I feel guilty, like I'm letting her die.

My mother was 91 when she was in a nursing home with Alzheimer's. I had DNR-cc papers drawn up for her years earlier but I never really had to use them. After my mother broke her hip, things began to get more complicated. Hospice was already working with my mother at the nursing home because she had a couple of episodes of vomiting blood due to ulcers in her stomach and esophagus. The doctor wanted to do more tests on my mother and was asking me to get DNR-arrest papers so that he could proceed.

I had seen my mother's panicked expression in the ambulance and emergency room and I didn't want her to go through that trauma again but

I also didn't want to avoid giving her whatever help she would need to get better.

I was torn between two decisions; do I let Mom come to a natural end to her life by consenting to comfort care only or give the doctor my stamp of approval to do whatever invasive testing or surgery he deemed necessary?

Since Mom wasn't able to make decisions for herself, I had to search my heart through prayer and consulting with the head nurse, my husband, brother and hospice worker. I finally decided to go with the DNR-cc, but you may decide differently.

The age of your parent, their health condition and the amount of finances to cover invasive procedures are all a part of the POAs decision-making process. Once you make your decision, don't look back.

Be assured that whatever DNR you choose, it will not cause your parent's death. Their age, that critical fall they had, their existing health problems and/or their poor health habits were all contributing factors.

A hundred years ago, you wouldn't have had to make these choices. There were no EMS workers, no living wills, no DNR papers or organ transplants to choose from. High tech times call for strong caregivers who must shoulder some challenging decisions, but guilt need not stifle you as a POA. Whatever you decide is the right decision.

Looking back on some of my decisions as POA, I wonder if I should have done what I did? Should I have changed doctors earlier? Should I have spent all that money on her room renovation?

Before you beat yourself into a guilt-ridden pulp, let me ask what you *did* do? Did you visit your parent? Did you get all the paperwork set up for them? Were you paying their bills or taking them to the doctor's office? Were you concerned about their health problems? I imagine you said yes to most or all of those things. And if you were to make a detailed list of all you did for your parent, I'm guessing it would take up a couple of pages or maybe a journal.

If the right decision were easy to see we wouldn't have so many choices. Invest in this company, not that. Go to this hospital, not that one. Who's right? Who's wrong?

Medical professionals often question if they did the right thing, but in the end, you only have to answer one question—"Did I try to do the best I could?" Stop obsessing over what others have done for their parent or, in hind sight, what you might have done differently for yours.

Somerset Maugham once wrote, "There is a sort of man who pays no attention to his good actions but is tormented by his bad ones." Don't be that tormented "sort of man" or woman. Appreciate what you have done and thank everyone who has helped you or your parent.

You might want to pick up an old recording of Bing Crosby and the Andrew Sisters that goes, "You've got to accentuate the positive, eliminate the negative, latch on to the affirmative, don't mess with mister-in-between." And I kinda think that *mister-in-between* had to be guilt.

CHAPTER 14
IMPORTANT: GETTING ORGANIZED

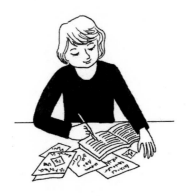

So now that you have lots of ideas and probably mounds of paperwork from your research, parent's important files and notes you've taken about your parent's health, thoughts and information—you need a way to keep it all together. That's exactly why I created this chapter.

If you record the information in this book, it will help keep your important caregiver stuff in one place.

Of course, you should retain the accordion file, mentioned earlier, for *copies* of the important papers (like the living will, POA papers, etc.) but this chapter should be able to give you the check lists of things needed to ask the estate lawyer, funeral director, financial planner, head nurse, doctor or the insurance agent.

You also may want to make copies of the following pages* (especially if you are caring for more than one person) and even enlarge them, so you can record your facts more easily. As long as you are using the pages for personal use for you or a family member, that is perfectly all right.

I suggest that you clearly print everything in PENCIL, since addresses, phone numbers and company names or policies may change. **And use a very fine lead** (accounting pencil), **so you can neatly squeeze in all the important details.**

I did not include a place for your parent's social security number, even though you will need it for various transactions. So you might want to memorize it, keep it in a safe place or write it inconspicuously in the margin of one of these pages. It's amazing what the wrong person can do with someone's social security number if they get a hold of it.

Also, you may make copies* of the pages in this chapter for your own personal use and keep them in your file and even give a copy* to the secondary POA and executor of your parent's estate. If you are caregiver to BOTH of your parents, you will probably want a copy of the following information for each parent.

So gather up all those Post-a-Notes and scribbled telephone messages and get ORGANIZED. And by the way, if you should run into terms, like TOD or DNR, that you're not sure of—check out chapter 8 for their definitions.

*This entire book has been copyrighted and can not be duplicated for any commercial reason in any form. However, you may copy the contents of chapter 14 for multiple individuals in your own family. For any other use of the material, you will need permission from the author, Donna Trickett at **www.donnatrickett.com**

VERY IMPORTANT

These are the most important pieces of paper my parent will need FROM:

the **Estate (Elder Care) Attorney:**

☐ A Last Will and Testament or Trust

☐ A Living Will

☐ Durable POA (Power of Attorney) papers over your parent's finances

☐ Durable POA (Power of Attorney) papers over your parent's health

the **Financial Advisor, Insurance Agent,** and **Bank:**

☐ Check that all financial investments and documents have a TOD clause.

the **Doctor** or **Nurse Practitioner:**

☐ DNR-cc or DNR-arrest

☐ Handicap tag for car visor (if applicable)

My parent needs to GIVE copies of the following documents to . . .

the Primary and Secondary POA:

☐ A Last Will and Testament or Trust

☐ A Living Will

☐ Durable POA (Power of Attorney) papers over your parent's finances

☐ Durable POA (Power of Attorney) papers over your parent's health

☐ DNR-cc or DNR-arrest

the Financial Advisor, Insurance Agent, CPA, and Bank:

☐ Durable POA (Power of Attorney) papers over your parent's finances

the Doctor, Nurse Practitioner, Hospital, or Head Nurse:

☐ DNR-cc or DNR-arrest

☐ Durable POA (Power of Attorney) papers over your parent's health

☐ A Living Will

☐ Completed and updated medical information charts on the following Medical Information pages.

PERSONAL—phone numbers and addresses   Page 1 of 9

The following is a list of all the important people in your parent's life: ALL doctors, lawyer, Insurance agents, Hospital, CPA, siblings, head nurse, good friends, etc.

NAME	ADDRESS	P=Phone C=Cell E=Email
		P C E
		P C E
		P C E
		P C E
		P C E
		P C E
		P C E
		P C E
		P C E

PERSONAL—phone numbers and addresses

NAME	ADDRESS	P=Phone C=Cell E=Email
		P C E
		P C E
		P C E
		P C E
		P C E
		P C E
		P C E
		P C E
		P C E

PERSONAL-Where is everything?

After each category, make a note of where the policy, account, or agreement can be found, and if it is an investment or insurance policy: name the company, type of policy, and any numbers associated with the policy or investment.

Banking (checking, savings, CDs)

_____

_____

_____

_____

_____

_____

_____

_____

Investments (IRA, mutual funds, personal purchases of stocks or bonds, etc.)

_____

_____

_____

_____

_____

_____

_____

Jewelry and precious metals (silverware, gold coins, bouillons, etc.)

_____

_____

_____

_____

_____

_____

_____

PERSONAL-Where is everything?

Vehicle, motorcycle, boat, camper, airplane, etc.

_____

_____

_____

_____

_____

_____

_____

_____

Antiques, collectables and vintage cars

_____

_____

_____

_____

_____

_____

_____

_____

Insurance (home, car, boat, umbrella, life, health—including Medicare) * _Note_ **_Insurance_** _section in this chapter._

_____

_____

_____

_____

_____

_____

_____

_____

PERSONAL-Where is everything?

Others

_____

_____

_____

_____

_____

_____

_____

_____

_____

_____

_____

_____

_____

_____

_____

_____

_____

_____

_____

_____

_____

_____

_____

_____

_____

_____

_____

_____

_____

_____

_____

_____

PERSONAL-Questions for Your Parent

Serious Questions (to help make decisions about end-time-issues and create a memorial)

What do you want to be remembered for?

_____

_____

_____

What would you like to tell your children and grandchildren?

_____

_____

_____

_____

_____

What are your best memories?

_____

_____

_____

_____

_____

_____

What is your favorite book and author?

_____

_____

_____

_____

What is your favorite music, composer, or performer?

_____

_____

_____

_____

_____

PERSONAL-Questions for Your Parent

Some of these questions may be a bit sensitive so don't ask them all at once and pick the time when you feel they are most open to them, like after a stay in the hospital.

How do you feel about invasive medical procedures (surgeries, life support . . .)?

_____

_____

_____

Do you have a doctor you are comfortable with?

_____

_____

_____

How do you feel about alternative medicine (chiropractic, homeopathic, herbal, acupuncture, acupressure . . .)?

_____

_____

_____

What do you think happens when we die?

_____

_____

_____

What are the biggest changes since you were young?

_____

_____

_____

_____

Do you consider these changes to be good or bad and why?

_____

_____

_____

PERSONAL-Questions for Your Parent   Page 8 of 9

What is your favorite color?

_____

What is your favorite flower?

_____

What is your favorite pet?

_____

What is your favorite hobby?

_____

What is your favorite sport?

_____

Do you like to sing?

_____

What is your favorite food or foods? (Helpful with ordering food for them in their facility)

_____

_____

_____

What is your least favorite food or foods?

_____

_____

_____

Where did you enjoy vacationing?

_____

What is your pet peeve?

_____

Do you like using a computer?

_____

PERSONAL-Questions for Your Parent

Do you like to exercise?

_____

Do you like the out-of-doors?

_____

Do you like birds and squirrels?

_____

Do you have an instrument you like to play? What?

_____

_____

Do you have things you like to collect? What?

_____

_____

_____

Do you like having visitors or more time to be alone and read?

_____

What's your favorite movie?

_____

_____

Who is your favorite actor?

_____

What kind of clothes do you like to wear? (Casual, smart casual, formal, glitzy?)

_____

_____

What size clothing do you wear?

_____

What size shoe do you wear?

_____

LEGAL: Estate (Elder Law) Lawyer
(Take this information to an estate lawyer to draw up the legal documents)

Last Will and Testament or Trust

Name, address, and phone number of parent:

_____

_____

_____

_____

This is a list of all the assets they want to include in the Will or Trust: *(home, car, business, antiques, etc. and any specific distribution of those assets.)*

_____

_____

_____

_____

_____

_____

_____

_____

The names of the children or pets that are still under my parent's care and the names of the guardian or designated location for these individuals:

_____

_____

_____

_____

This is the person that my parent wants omitted from the Will.

_____

_____

_____

_____

LEGAL: Estate (Elder Law) Lawyer   Page 2 of 2
(Take this information to an estate lawyer to draw up the legal documents)

These are the beneficiaries my parent wants in their Will: **Primary beneficiaries** *(usually spouse or children):*

_____

_____

_____

_____

Secondary beneficiaries *(usually children or grandchildren):*

_____

_____

_____

_____

This is the name, address and phone number of the **primary executor** or **trustee** they have chosen to carry out their Will or Trust:

_____

_____

_____

_____

This is the name, address and phone number of the **alternate executor** or **trustee** they have chosen to carry out their Will or Trust:

_____

_____

_____

_____

Any additional information:

_____

_____

_____

_____

* Keep in mind that the more detailed the Will, the more costly the lawyer's fee.

INSURANCE:

Check that your parent has or considers adding insurance coverage in the following areas and then list the name of the company, the type policy, and the number of the policy:

House or Apartment (not normally required in assisted living or nursing home):

_____

_____

Personal Umbrella insurance:

_____

_____

Car or truck:

_____

Recreational vehicles (camper, aircraft, boat, motorcycle, etc.):

_____

_____

Business (if they own a business other than from the home):

_____

_____

Commercial Umbrella insurance:

_____

Long Term Care:

_____

_____

Medigap or Medicare supplement:

_____

_____

Final expense or funeral insurance (if not with funeral home):

_____

Life Insurance (whole or term):

_____

MEDICAL: Medical Information updated:_____   **Page 1 of 6**
(Keep updated monthly and after medical condition changes)

Patient's name: _____

Address: _____

_____

Home Phone: _____ Cell Phone: _____

Business Phone: _____ Email: _____

Date of Birth: _____

PRIMARY Insurance Company: _____

Policy Number: _____

Address and/or Phone number of above Primary Insurance Company:

_____

_____

SECONDARY Insurance Company: _____

Policy Number: _____

Address and/or Phone number of Secondary Insurance Company:

_____

_____

Additional Insurance Company: _____

Policy Number: _____

Address and/or Phone number of Additional Insurance Company:

_____

_____

Additional Insurance Company: _____

Policy Number: _____

Address and/or Phone number of Additional Insurance Company:

_____

_____

MEDICAL: Medical Information updated:_____   **Page 2 of 6**
(Keep updated monthly and after medical condition changes)

Doctor's name, type of practice (MD, OS, DDS) address and phone:

Doctor's name & Practice	Address	Phone
_____	_____	_____
_____	_____	_____
_____	_____	_____
_____	_____	_____
_____	_____	_____
_____	_____	_____

Who is official primary POA over the health of this patient?
Name: _____Phone: _____
Cell Phone: _____ Business Phone: _____

Who is official secondary POA over the health of this patient?
Name: _____ Phone: _____
Cell Phone: _____ Business Phone: _____
Durable POA over Health papers are located where?_____
_____

Who else can we call in an emergency?
Name: _____ (relationship): _____
Phone: _____
Cell Phone: _____ Business Phone: _____
Name: _____ (relationship): _____
Phone: _____
Cell Phone: _____ Business Phone: _____

Location of living will: _____
Are they an organ donor? ☐ YES or ☐ NO
Location of DNR papers: _____
Indicate which DNR designation: ☐ DNR-cc or ☐ DNR-arrest?

Definition of DNR designations can be found under the medical section in the dictionary chapter 8.

MEDICAL: Medical Information updated:_____
(Keep updated monthly and after medical condition changes)

MEDICAL ALERTS (implants, anticoagulants, epilepsy, etc.):

_____

_____

_____

_____

_____

_____

MEDICAL PROBLEMS (heart condition, hypertension, etc.)

_____

_____

_____

_____

_____

_____

ALLERGIES (to medications or surroundings):

_____

_____

_____

_____

_____

_____

MEDICATIONS: (present medications including vitamins)

_____

_____

_____

_____

_____

_____

MEDICAL: Medical Information updated:_____
(Keep updated monthly and after medical condition changes)

Patient's name: _____

Surgery, Accident, Illness	Date	Town & State

MEDICAL: Medical Information updated:_____

(Keep updated monthly and after medical condition changes)
Note inherent medical problems, like heart disease and, diabetes, not accidents or illnesses. Also, if a family member is deceased, print age and cause of death.

Patient's name:

_____

Birth Mother's name and medical history:

_____
_____
_____
_____

Grandmother's name and medical history on the **mother's** side:

_____
_____
_____
_____

Grandfather's name and medical history on the **mother's** side:

_____
_____
_____
_____

Birth Father's name and medical history:

_____
_____
_____
_____

Grandmother's name and medical history on the **father's** side:

_____
_____
_____
_____

MEDICAL: Medical Information updated:_____   Page 6 of 6
(Keep updated monthly and after medical condition changes)

Grandfather's name and medical history on the **father's** side:

_____

_____

_____

_____

_____

_____

Brothers and Sisters' names and medical history (not siblings from a step parent's family or adopted siblings):

_____

_____

_____

_____

_____

Aunts or Uncle's names and medical history:

_____

_____

_____

_____

_____

_____

The CHART on the following page is For YOUR RECORDS:
Make several copies if your parent has more medications or vitamins and keep updated

(Remember, vitamins can effect medications)

Medications and Vitamins for: _____   **Updated:** _____

Name of Medication	Dosage	What is it for?	Possible Side effects	Cost	Refill Date

How to draw up a MEDICATION INFORMATION letter
to the head nurse or nurse practitioner, if you are in charge of getting meds for your parent, (keep the FAX or make copies of any letters, in case there is a question later):

Jane Smith daughter and POA for Mary Smith
5555 Happy Lane; Happy Valley, MD 55555
555-555-5555 JS@ihavemail.net

January 10, 2009

Happy Valley Nursing Home
Attention: Susan Jones, RN
345 Shady Lane Dr.
Happy Valley, MD 55555

Dear Susan,

According to my records, we will be meeting with you on Tuesday, January 16 at 10 a.m. Also, in accordance with our last meeting, I had nurse Johnson sign for the following medications that I dropped off this morning, January 10:

     Protonix, 40 mg., which should be good until March 10
     Isosorbide 60 mg., which should be good until March 10

I understand that I will continue to be responsible for the following medications and vitamin renewals as they run out:

     Celexa 20 mg.
     Protonix 40 mg.
     Multiple vitamin

Hospice Vista Care will be supplying :

     Lactulose 30cc
     Risperdal 1 mg.

And the following medications have been dropped:

     Miacalcin Nasal Spray

Thank you for your continued care and attention to my mother's needs.

Sincerely,
Jane Smith POA for Mary Smith

Letter of Introduction to Nursing Home Facility

This informal letter is not required but it does make the transition easier on your parent and the staff. Include early and recent pictures of your parent:

Name: _____

Name of spouse: _____

Is spouse living or dead? _____ When did they die? _____

Names of children (designate M=male, F=female, L=living or D=deceased)

_____

_____

_____

_____

Names of siblings (designate M=male, F=female, L=living or D=deceased)

_____

_____

_____

_____

Career or jobs she once had: _____

_____

Hobbies she has enjoyed: _____

_____

Activities** that she once participated in, such as skiing, boating, etc. : _____

_____

_____

Places she has traveled to: _____

_____

Places**she lived: _____

_____

Food preferences: _____

_____

Food allergies or dislikes: _____

_____

HOUSING-Out of Their Home

This check list will help you to decide whether your parent should remain alone or if they need a visiting nurse or change their housing to your home or consider other choices.

☐ Is their bedroom, bath, and living area on the first floor?

☐ Is the entrance to the house manageable for their condition? (single step with railing or ramp)

☐ Are they still able to drive a car, and if not, do they have public or private means of transportation to get them to the store and doctor?

☐ Are they eating properly? Check their refrigerator and cupboards.

☐ Are they taking their medications on time? Consider labeled pill dispensers.

☐ Can your parent safely and easily dress and bathe? Do they need handrails next to the toilet and around the tub or shower?

☐ Is there a capable adult living with them, such as a healthy spouse?

☐ Is your parent suffering from depression (bipolar) Alzheimer's or dementia, severe heart issues, and/or physical or mental handicaps? You might want to consider a more vigilant care facility.

☐ Does your parent have a medical alert device on their person or easily accessible in their house, in case of an emergency?

☐ Are the hallways and furnishings giving enough room for them to get around easily and safely?

☐ Is the house kept reasonably clean and uncluttered?

☐ Is your parent open to the idea of a visiting nurse or live-in hired caregiver?

HOUSING-Out of YOUR Home

Approximate cost: $500-$1500/mon. **

Extra expenses for a ramp, bathroom alterations, hospital bed, and/or a visiting nurse—as well as living expenses could cost you $500 to $1500/month, which could be covered by your parent's Social Security and IRA withdrawals. Look over other considerations below:

☐ Is the entrance to your house manageable for their condition? (single step with railing or ramp)

☐ Will you be available to drive them to the store and doctor appointments?

☐ Can you provide them with nutritious meals, according to their medical needs (low salt, low sugar, low fat) throughout the day?

☐ Are you able to check that they take their meds, possibly at three specific times throughout the day?

☐ Are you able to help them dress and bathe?

☐ Is your parent suffering from depression (bipolar) Alzheimer's or dementia, severe heart issues, and/or physical or mental handicaps—and do you feel qualified to care for them, physically and knowledgably?

☐ Does your parent have a medical alert device on their person or easily accessible in your house, in case of an emergency?

☐ Are the hallways and furnishings giving enough room for them to get around easily and safely?

☐ Is the house kept reasonably clean and uncluttered?

☐ Do you have unruly pets that could trip them or push them down?

☐ Is their bedroom and bath on the first floor?

☐ Is your parent open to the idea of a visiting nurse or live-in hired caregiver?

☐ Is your parent open to staying in an Adult Day Care occasionally? (Which could cost up to $150/day**.)

**housing statistics according to 2009 findings of www.aplaceformom.com

HOUSING-Retirement Community

Approximate cost: $1000-$3000/mon. **

☐ Is the community within an hour of your residence?

☐ Is your parent able to manage on their own? (cooking, cleaning . . .) If not, the community should have a room and board apartment option.

☐ Does the community provide a Life Care option, if your parent runs out of money?

☐ Do they have an Out Option, if they decide to move to another retirement community in a few years?

☐ What all is included in this monthly bill? Electric, water, gas, cable, free regular health checks, local phone service, weekly maid service?

☐ Does the facility allow for pets?

☐ Does the facility have an emergency signal to alert the on-duty nurse to give them assistance? (button or taking phone off the receiver)

☐ Do the workers at the community seem friendly and helpful?

☐ Do the present residents seem to enjoy their home and campus?

☐ Does the community offer a wide selection of housing options?

☐ Does the campus include assisted living and nursing home facility?

☐ Have you checked out the assisted living and nursing home portion of the community? Does it look like a good place for your parent if they should need that level of care?

☐ If your parent likes gardening, do they have a resident's garden area?

☐ Are the surroundings pleasant and well maintained?

☐ Are the sidewalks and roads in good condition and adequate in elevation and distance to activities to give your parent exercise on foot or by bike?

☐ Do they have an on campus Bank? Chapel? Library? Cafeteria for company or snacking? A formal dining hall for residents and parties? Grocery store for small provisions? Beauty or barber shop? Exercise room? Woodworking shop? Craft area?

☐ Does the facility have transportation to activities and shopping?

☐ Does the facility have a swimming pool and/or Jacuzzi?

☐ Are there free entertainment nights?

☐ Can your parent have a garage for their Car? Camper? Boat?

**housing statistics according to 2009 findings of www.aplaceformom.com

HOUSING-Assisted Living

Approximate cost: $2000-$4000/mon.** doctors & medication not included

This list will help you to decide if it's time to consider assisted living and how to choose the right one. It's not mandatory, but often suggested by a nurse or doctor.

- [ ] Does your parent suffer from Alzheimer's or dementia?
- [ ] Are they physically or mentally incapable of managing their everyday needs, such as cooking, cleaning, bathing, dressing, etc.?
- [ ] Is the facility within an hour of your home?*
- [ ] Is the facility certified? Check CareScout® unbiased ratings and reviews of facilities.
- [ ] Is the facility clean?
- [ ] Do the residents seem to enjoy it there?
- [ ] Are there plenty of activities to interest your parent? *(There should be a schedule of the week's activities posted.)*
- [ ] Tour the assisted living facility several times, before deciding. The age or attractiveness of a facility isn't as important as the quality of care and interaction between the staff and the residents. (If your parent is moving into a retirement community, check out the assisted living facility on the campus before signing the contract, even before they need the facility.)
- [ ] Be sure to have a long talk with any concerned family members or friends, who may not agree with your decision. A negative sibling or friend's visit can lead to a disgruntled parent who may want to leave, when it's not in their best interest.
- [ ] Consider making the room homey for your parent. *(note chapter 10 & 11)*
- [ ] Don't think because your parent is cared for that you don't need to visit as much. Patients who get more visitors get better care from the staff.
- [ ] It's nice to have the assisted living on the same retirement campus they enjoyed living in for several years, because they will have more friends to visit and share activities with.
- [ ] Is there a family counseling session with the staff so that you can better assess your parent's needs and progress?
- [ ] How is personal laundry handled? Is that an additional charge?
- [ ] How are pharmacy bills paid? *(You may want to get discount meds, see medical chart on previous page.)*

**housing statistics according to 2009 findings of www.aplaceformom.com

HOUSING-Nursing Home
Approximate cost: $4000-$8000/mon.**doctors & medications not included

☐ Does your parent have Alzheimer's or dementia and are roaming? (How will your parent be monitored? Bracelet alarm or door alarm?)

☐ Are they physically or mentally incapable of managing their everyday needs, and require constant nurses' attention?

☐ Is the facility within an hour of your home?

☐ Is the facility certified? Check CareScout® unbiased ratings and reviews of facilities.

☐ Is the facility clean?

☐ Do the residents seem to enjoy it there?

☐ Are there plenty of activities to interest your parent? (There should be a schedule of the week's activities posted and they should have outings scheduled to take residents on trips or to the store.)

☐ Tour the nursing home facility several times before deciding. The age or attractiveness of a facility isn't as important as the quality of care and interaction between the staff and the residents. (If your parent is moving into a retirement community, check out the nursing home facility on the campus before signing the contract, even before they need the facility.)

☐ Be sure to have a long talk with any concerned family members or friends, who may not agree with your decision. A negative sibling or friend's visit can lead to a disgruntled parent who may want to leave, when it's not in their best interest.

☐ Consider all the ways you can make the room more enjoyable for your parent. (note chapter 10 and 11)

☐ Don't think that because your parent is cared for, you don't need to visit as much. Truth is patients who get more visitors get better care from the staff.

☐ It's nice to have the nursing home on the same retirement campus they enjoyed living in for several years, because they will have more friends to visit and share activities with.

☐ Is there a family counseling session with the staff?

☐ How is personal laundry handled? Is there an additional charge?

☐ How are pharmacy bills paid? (You may want to get discount meds, see medical chart on previous page.)

**housing statistics according to 2009 findings of www.aplaceformom.com

HOUSING-Residential Care   **Page 6 of 6**
Approximate cost: $1500-$3000/mon.**

If the above housing options seem too expensive or just not what you want for your parent, there are a wide variety of Personal Care Homes or what is called Residential Care Homes, which are private homes usually with a smaller number of patients. Adult caretakers live at the facility but are not necessarily a professional medical person. The advantage is a more home-like community atmosphere.

☐ Not appropriate for Alzheimer's or dementia patients, especially when they begin to roam.

☐ Not appropriate for the physically or mentally handicapped who require constant nurses' attention.

☐ Is the facility within an hour of your home?*

☐ Is the facility certified?

☐ Is the facility clean?

☐ Do the residents seem to enjoy it there?

☐ Do you feel comfortable with the amount of medical attention they offer?

☐ Are there plenty of activities to interest your parent? (There should be a schedule of the week's activities posted and they should have outings scheduled to take residents on trips or to the store.)

☐ Is there a family counseling session with the staff?

☐ How is personal laundry handled? Is there an additional charge?

☐ How are pharmacy bills paid? (You may want to get discount meds, see medical chart on previous page.)

HOUSING-Hospice Facility

In order to use the hospice facility in your area, your parent must qualify. It is an end-of-life facility and not a place for a wheelchair or Alzheimer's patient who may require years of assistance and care because of their non-life-threatening circumstance. Check with your local hospice facility to see if your parent qualifies and by all means, if they do qualify, take advantage of hospice's exceptional care.

**housing statistics according to 2009 findings of www.aplaceformom.com

FUNERAL-Check List

Explain to your parent: "*I know it may seem a bit uncomfortable to talk about funerals, but I want to know what you want so I can carry out your wishes.*"

☐ Name, address and phone number of funeral home** you prefer:

_____

_____

☐ Have you preplanned your funeral with the funeral home?

_____

_____

☐ Have you PRE-PAID your funeral with the funeral home?

_____

_____

**Even though, you may have prepaid your funeral and many of the following questions were probably covered by the funeral home, please answer them again, so I know your wishes.

☐ Do you have a burial plot? _____ If so, where is it located, who do I need to contact and where is the deed to the plot?

_____

_____

☐ Do you already have a headstone in place? _____ If not, what kind would you like and how would you like it to read?

_____

_____

Possible funeral services:

☐ Traditional Funeral service: funeral home service to internment service.
☐ One viewing on two separate days, followed by funeral service?
☐ One early viewing followed by funeral service on the same day?
☐ Cremation with memorial service in funeral home with later burial of ashes in cemetery or dispersing the ashes in the place of your parent's choice. (This can be done days or months after their cremation)
☐ A rented casket for a traditional funeral service followed by cremation.
☐ If your parent can not afford the above choices or does not want an elaborate funeral, they may opt to be cremated and have a simple memorial service out of their church, home, or at a significant site where they want their ashes to be distributed.

FUNERAL-Check List

Traditional Funeral details:

**Name, address, and phone number or clergyman you prefer:

_____

_____

_____

_____

Preference of casket style, color, etc. _____

_____

**Name, address, and phone number of any special musician you prefer to sing or play at your funeral, as well as the tune you want them to perform:

_____

_____

**Name music, scripture or poems you want heard at your funeral:

_____

_____

Cremation Options (may include items** from above list):

Is there a special day that you would like the burial ceremony of the ashes and what cemetery have you picked? _____

If not a cemetery burial, is there a special place you would want the ashes scattered? _____

_____

Do you want a traditional funeral service with rented casket, then cremation and dispersing of the ashes after the funeral? _____

_____

Do you have any particular preferences as to the urn that you prefer?

_____

_____

Other:

_____

_____

FUNERAL-Check List   **Page 3 of 6**

**Do you or have you belonged to any special groups, organizations, or military service that you would like to acknowledge at your funeral? Please include any contact people and phone numbers:

_____

_____

_____

_____

_____

_____

What are your favorite flowers and color of those flowers?

_____

_____

Do you have a favorite charity you would like friends and family to give to instead of sending flowers? _____

_____

_____

Do you have a preference as to the clothing, jewelry, etc. to be buried in? _____
If yes, can you describe it: _____

_____

_____

**Do you wish to leave any personal letters or videos for your children or grandchildren? _____ If yes, have they been made yet? _____ If yes, where can I find them?

_____

_____

_____

_____

** Be sure to contact the above people to be sure they are willing to give their services and then be sure to contact them as soon as you believe your parent is in a serious health condition. And try to gather the musical CDs, DVDs, scriptures, and poems as early as possible, and put them in a file in your home.

FUNERAL-Obituary   **Page 4 of 6**

You may compose your own obituary or just supply the paper with the following for them to put together. Omit any information you would rather not have included.

In which newspapers would you want to announce your parent's passing? *(Consider hometown, their present resident campus paper, your local paper. Funeral homes will usually get the obituary out to the newspaper of your choosing if you let them know their name, email and/or phone number.)*

_____

_____

_____

Include photo for newspaper (optional).

Parent's full name: _____

Date of death: _____

Age at time of death: _____

What was the cause of death? _____

Where did they die? _____

What was their job or profession? _____

What high school or college did they attend and what degree did they acquire?

_____

_____

What branch of the military did they serve in, their rank and which war?

_____

_____

Name of organizations, church, clubs, or volunteer work they participated in:

_____

_____

Names of close relatives who survived them *(spouse, siblings, children, grandchildren, great grandchildren).*

_____

_____

_____

_____

_____

_____

FUNERAL-Obituary

You may prefer to just give the numbers instead of the names of all the relatives:

☐ Number of siblings: _____
☐ Number of children: _____
☐ Number of grandchildren: _____
☐ Number of great grandchildren: _____
☐ Name, location and directions to funeral home (include a map):

_____
_____
_____
_____
_____

☐ Time and day or days of viewings

_____
_____
_____
_____
_____

☐ Time and day of funeral

_____
_____
_____
_____

☐ Preferences for donations to an organization instead of flowers (give name and phone number or contact address):

_____
_____
_____
_____

FUNERAL-Memorial Bulletin (optional)

Here is a copy of the bulletin I made for my mother's funeral. You can purchase decorative paper for funerals from a print shop or you can accept the bulletin offered by the funeral home.

Anyone who knew my mother knew that she had a joyful spirit of giving and caring. Even though Alzheimer's had dimmed her thoughts, Mom never stopped smiling or being thankful. She would often thank the nurses for her evening pills and ask if we wanted to share the food on her tray.

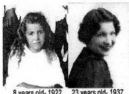

8 years old- 1922   23 years old- 1937   85 years old- 1999

Alice Olga Killip
1914-2005

Born at home in Donora, PA as the third of nine surviving brothers and sisters, my mother's family later moved to a small farm in Cambridge, OH. Her father, Felix Parry, died when she was fifteen, so she had to work as a maid and waitress in order to help support the family during the Great Depression.

She and my Dad, Donald, eloped to Niagara Falls in 1937. Dad was drafted into the army and served in the occupation of Japan from 1945 to 1946. Mom managed financially by sewing aprons and cleaning houses, while caring for my brother, Bill, and I.

After raising their children, Mom and Dad got a sailboat, *Whispering Hope*, and later a camper. They visited the magnificent Grand Canyon, danced at their grandson's wedding in Albuquerque, took pictures of the grandeur of Yosemite, and had peaceful sailing trips with their grandchildren to Cedar Point. As Dad's health declined, they moved into an apartment in Copeland Oaks. Mom served him faithfully for 9 years through his many surgeries and medical needs. Dad died at 80 and they were married almost 60 yrs.

Mom always found some means of making extra money. When she was 81, she created her own little business making kitchen hand towels to sell at the Acorn Shop. Unfortunately, when she turned 87, Mom was diagnosed with Alzheimer's and needed to move into an assisted living apartment. Her continued decline in health mandated her move to Crandal Nursing Home.

When my husband, Nelson, and I moved to Columbus, Ohio to be with our son, his wife, and our first grandchild ...we moved Mom to a neighboring nursing home and had many enjoyable visits and trips together.

When she went through a trying experience in the hospital in 2004, she turned to me and said, "I'm sorry to put you through all this." Not..."Get me out of here"...but "I'm sorry to put you through all this." And after having not had any liquids for over 24 hours, when she was dying of thirst, a nurse offered her a glass of cold water and Mom asked Nelson and I if we would like some. Recently, after recovering from a broken hip, when I asked how she was, she said, "I'm fine and how are you doing?" Her continuous love and generous ways will remain in my heart forever.

Written with loving memories by her daughter...Donna Trickett

Alice is survived by **TWO children**, Bill Killip and his wife, Carol; **Donna Trickett** and her husband, Nelson; **THREE grandsons**, Scott Killip and his wife Cindy, Eric Killip and his wife Jackie, and Kirk Trickett and his wife Sabrina; and **SIX great grandchildren**: Laura and Andy Killip, Benjamin and Brooklyn Killip, and Joseph and Savanna Trickett; **ONE brother**, Steve Parry and his wife Anne, and **ONE sister** Betty Walter and her husband Jim.

Her husband, Donald and one granddaughter, Kimberly Trickett, preceded her in death.

Things to do BEFORE your parent dies

If your parent is critically ill:
Many of the asterisk items below can be kept in your accordion file so that you don't have to search when your time could be better spent in other matters.

- [ ] Alert family & friends* *(Names and phone numbers on previous pages.)*
- [ ] Alert funeral director*
- [ ] Ask for up to 10 death certificates *(for closing important accounts)*
- [ ] Alert special music performer*
- [ ] Alert clubs, organization, or military service*
- [ ] Locate will or trust*
- [ ] Locate deed to cemetery plot*
- [ ] Locate scriptures or poems*
- [ ] Locate special music requests*
- [ ] Locate your parents special letters or videos*
- [ ] Locate a photo of your parent for the funeral director to use when preparing your parent for viewing and for obituary.*
- [ ] Pick out the clothing your parent will wear for their funeral *(You often can leave it with the funeral home a year or more in advance.)*
- [ ] Put together copies of old photos to display at the funeral *(Good if you can have a note next to each picture to describe what it represents; place, age, etc. Also, having them in chronological order makes more sense to the viewer.)*
- [ ] Put together a eulogy, a tribute to be read at the funeral.
- [ ] Put together a program for the funeral; who will do what and when.
- [ ] Create an obituary (note previous pages) and decide what papers to put it in. (Newspapers often charge for obituary announcements.)
- [ ] Create a memorial bulletin to be given out at the funeral home. (note the previous pages) By the way, funeral homes do offer a stock bulletin with your choice of wording and a couple of facts about your parent, if you prefer.

Immediately AFTER your parent's death   **Page 1 of 3**

*These duties should be done by the **executor** or **trustee** of your parent's Will or Trust. And it's a good idea to give a copy of the information to the secondary executor. Keep copies of all FAX and email transactions.*

CALL the following: *(keep the conversations brief, and explain that you have a lot to do and will spend time talking or in a letter, after the funeral).*
HOSPICE, if you have been working with them:

_____

FUNERAL HOME

_____

_____

CONTRACTED Funeral Home** *(That's the funeral home where your parent's funeral will be held, which may be different from the funeral home that picked up the body of your parent after their death):*

_____

_____

**Review agreed upon details of funeral by fax or email directives. The funeral home should order flowers and take care of other details.
**Let the funeral home know the day and times you want for the viewing and funeral. *(Consider the distances some of the bereaved will have to travel)*
FAX or email obituary notice to funeral home and request that they send out obituary notices to newspapers of your choosing, noted in the **Funeral: Obituary section in this chapter.
**Request up to 10 death certificates from the Funeral Home.
CLERGYMAN. _____
Person doing SPECIAL MUSIC. _____

EXECUTOR, if you're not the one named in the will.

_____

_____

Your SURVIVING PARENT, even if they were divorced, if they haven't already been notified. (They probably want to see them for the last time, so allow them private time.)

_____

_____

Immediately AFTER your parent's death

CALL the following:

Your BROTHERS and SISTERS (Including half, adopted, or foster siblings. Ask them to call their children . . . your parent's grandchildren . . . even if you want to talk to everyone, there is too much to do right now and you need their help.):

_____

_____

_____

_____

_____

_____

_____

_____

_____

Your PARENT'S BROTHERS and SISTERS, living parents and close family members.

_____

_____

_____

_____

_____

_____

_____

_____

_____

_____

_____

Immediately AFTER your parent's death

CALL the following:

Close friends in their facility, neighbors, cousins, or church friends:

_____

_____

_____

_____

_____

_____

_____

_____

Any close friends of yours that you want to notify

_____

_____

_____

_____

_____

_____

_____

_____

Finish the following:

- [ ] Putting together a picture board. (optional)
- [ ] Putting together the memorial bulletin. (optional)
- [ ] Putting together your outfit. Black is traditional, but most of all, it needs to respect your parent.
- [ ] Arrange for private room in restaurant for immediate family or friends, after the internment. (Or, if you have a church or group who will arrange for a snack or meal at the church or other facility after the internment, that's great, too.)

Within a WEEK after your parent's death

*Remember, you must be the **executor** of your parent's will in order to carry out the duties AFTER your parent's death. **Save all information for six years after their death.***

Call the **BANK** to find out how much was in your parent's account at the time of their death. _____

Give **BANK** an original death certificate.

> If you had a joint account, keep accurate records of the amount in the account at the time of death and AFTER paying bills, then divide the remaining money according to the will. (Don't settle the estate too quickly, lingering doctor and hospital bills could take months to finalize, and if it goes into probate, it could take a year.)

Call **FINANCIAL ADVISOR** to find out how much was in their account at the time of their death. _____

Give **FINANCIAL ADVISOR** an original death certificate.

Call the **ESTATE LAWYER** to tell him the total sum of your parent's estate at the time of death, so he can prepare a tax statement. _____

Give **ESTATE LAWYER** an original death certificate.

ESTATE LAWYER may require a reading of the will.

Call the **INSURANCE AGENT** _____

Give the **INSURANCE AGENT** an original death certificate.

Call SOCIAL SECURITY _____

Cancel your parent's social security number so it cannot be used fraudulently.

Send an original death certificate to **SOCIAL SECURITY.**

Call **MEDICARE** (Medigap or Medicare Part C and/or Medicaid)

_____

Send original death certificate to **MEDICARE** or other insurance programs.

Contact any other insurance coverage: *Send original death certificate to each one.*

_____

_____

Call any other pension, investment, or income group. *Send another death certificate to each of them.*

_____

_____

Others:

_____

_____

Additional Information:

CHAPTER 15
RESOURCE MATERIAL

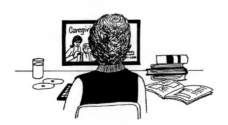

Contact **Area Agency on Aging** at **www.n4a.org** or call 1-800-677-1116 for all kinds of help connecting your parent to a variety of services in your area.

Ask.com, at **www.ask.com** and **Google.com** at **www.google.com** are great ways to get a lot of quick answers to just about any questions. Just type in your question and it will pick out the key words to locate a host of websites that you can check out.

BOOKS
If a book is out of print, check a secondhand bookstore or Amazon.com

DEALING with DEATH:

Compassion Books, Inc. is a group who has found over 400 books, videos and audios to help children and adults through serious illness, death and dying, grief, bereavement and losses of all kinds, including divorce, suicide, trauma, sudden loss and violence. You will definitely want to check out **www.compassionbooks.com**

ALZHEIMER'S:

Inside Mom's Mind, Journey into the thoughts of an Alzheimer's patient **by Donna M. Trickett.** Xlibris Corporation. 2008. This is the true story of the author's caregiving experience, riddled with moments of frustration, laughter, confusion and inspiration. You will experience the mental decline and ever-changing emotions of her mother by actually listening into her thought process. As a bonus, Donna has created a help section in the back of the book along with helpful ideas throughout the story that will give you over 100 ways to better understand the disease and make the journey more enjoyable for you and your parent. **www.donnatrickett.com**

Elder Rage, Take My Father . . . Pease! **by Jacqueline Marcell.** Impressive Press. 2001. Jacqueline shares the frustration and humor of taking care of a not-so-docile parent in the throes of Alzheimer's. The graphic images and language are quite strong, but if you have a very difficult situation with your parent, this may help you know you're not alone and give you lots of ideas and resources for dealing with your situation. Jacqueline also hosts an internet radio talk show for caregivers called *Coping with Caregiving* on **wsradio.com** which discusses a variety of topics related to the issues of the caregiver. Just go to the website (www.wsradio.com) and click on "health, mind, and body" and then click on "Coping with Caregiving" to hear past interviews with authors and experts in the field.

The 36-Hour Day, A Family Guide to Caring for People with Alzheimer's Disease, Other Dementias, and Memory Loss in Later Life **by Ms. Nancy L. Mace MA, Dr. Peter V. Rabins MD MPh, and Dr. Paul R. McHugh MD.** Baltimore: A John Hopkins Press Health Book. 2006 An extremely thorough study of Alzheimer's and dementia by this team of doctors brings awareness to the issues and feelings of the patient as well as detailed analysis of their needed care. If you really want to understand what your dementia parent is experiencing and why, this book will cover all the aspects that you may not have been able to understand before.

CAREGIVING:

Caregiving 101, with 1001 easy-to-understand bits of vital information **by Donna M. Trickett.** Xlibris Corporation. 2011. This is a must have for any caregiver. It will help you through the basics of the legal, medical, financial, guilt and spiritual matters that face you and your parent in the end-of-life issues. A no-nonsense dictionary will help you understand the legal, medical and financial jargon. Helpful charts, vital records, housing options, crafts and activities to help your aging patient, insightful chapters on aging issues will all serve to help make you a more compassionate and confident caregiver. This book is not only a necessary resource *for* the caregiver to have but it's a great gift *from* the parent to their caregiver. **www.donnatrickett.com**

Caregiver's Handbook: A Complete Guide to Home Health Care by **Visiting Nurses Associations of America**. DK Publishing. 1998. If you are planning to take care of your parent out of your home, temporarily or permanently, this is a must have book.

CHILDREN'S BOOKS ABOUT SENIORS:

Often young children and teens are deeply affected by the thought of losing their grandparent, or even great grandparent, to a nursing home, Alzheimer's or death. They may not be able to talk about their feelings and that's where these books can be very helpful.

After the Funeral by **Jane Loretta**. Winsch-Paulist Press 1995. Through the honest words of several bereaved children who have lost a mother, father, grandparent, sibling, or friend; the adult reader can help their child understand his hurt, fear, anger or embarrassment.

Grandfather and I by **Helen E. Buckley**. Lothrop Publishing. 1994. Appreciating the fact that grandpas take the time to enjoy things because they slow down, this book follows an African American grandfather with his grandson as they enjoy a nature walk together with some storytelling time.

Grandma According to Me by **Karen Magnuson Beil**. Doubleday Publishing. 1992. This is a delightfully illustrated and positive book about a young granddaughter's enjoyment of her grandparents, particularly her grandmother. It helps a child appreciate the signs of aging, such as wrinkles, as a sign of love.

I'll See You In My Dreams by **Stacey Schuett**. Knopf Publishing. 2002. This book is about a little girl who flies on an airline to visit her dying uncle who was a pilot but is now in a nursing home. She dreams of writing messages in the sky to him and then has to face the reality of his new surroundings. This book helps a child accept a loved one in a hospital or nursing home.

Poppy's Chair by **Karen Hesse.** Scholastic Publishing. 2000. After the death of Leah's grandfather, she comes to stay with her grandmother for two weeks. She and her grandmother reminisce about Poppy and enjoy sitting in his chair.

Remember That by **Leslea Newman.** Clarion Books. 1993. This story shows how a Jewish grandmother has taught her granddaughter the traditions of her faith through her words and actions. The book takes you through several declining years with Bubbe, as grandma is called. Bubbe becomes weaker and eventually goes into a nursing home where they still maintain a relationship and grandma still reminds her granddaughter of her life-lessons with her favorite phrase, "Remember that."

The Next Place by **Warren Hanson.** Waldman house Press Inc. 1997. This book creates a rather vague yet beautiful image of what heaven will be like. The author has used words and inspiring images that do not depict any particular religion and yet give hope to the young reader. I used this book to help encourage my 91-year-old Alzheimer's mother as she remained in bed in the last crucial days of her life. It made her smile.

FINANCIAL:

The Wall Street Journal, Guide to Understanding Personal Finance by **Kenneth M. Morris and Alan M. Siegel.** Lightbulb Press, Inc. 1998. It's an easy-read colorful and accurate way to pick up some quick savvy about you and your parent's finances. Other titles by the Wall Street Journal are: **_Guide to Planning Your Financial Future, the Easy-to-Read Guide to Planning for Retirement_** and **_Guide to Understanding Money & Investing._**

INTERNET CONNECTIONS

ELDER CARE ISSUES:

AARP. The American Association of Retired Persons. Go to: **www.aarp.org** to learn more about AARP membership, discounts and informative magazines. They can help your parent locate doctors and lawyers, too.

Alzheimer's Association of America. www.alz.org is filled with information to help you locate a facility for your parent and understand more about the care of your parent. They also provide educational workshops, support groups and FREE weekly enews letters to keep you informed about the disease.

Alzheimer's Foundation of America. www.alzfdn.org is the website for the Alzheimer's Foundation of America. It's filled with information about medical findings, caregiving, and offers a free magazine with helpful information, called *Care ADvantage*.

Brokers and Investment Advisors. When you go to **www.sec.gov/investor/ brokers.htm** you will be on the U.S. Securities and Exchange Commissions website. This particular link will help you understand in more detail what to look for in a financial advisor and even give you a place to check out the company and advisor's status.

Care Scout. www.carescout.com is CareScout®'s website for unbiased housing facility searches for the elderly.

Eldercare Link. www.eldercarelink.com will help you find eldercare in your state.

Hospice. www.hospicenet.org for information about hospice and local hospice chapters near you.

Medicare. www.medicare.com, www.medicare.org, and **www.medicare.gov** for all your Medicare questions, including various coverages that are available.

Medicaid. www.medicaid.com and **www.medicaid.org** for all your Medicaid questions, including what are the requirements for being eligible for Medicaid.

National Association of Professional Geriatric Care Managers NAPGCM **www.caremanager.org** may be able to guide you through a plan of care for your parent.

National Church Residences. www.ncr.org for low to moderate housing and medical care facilities for seniors.

A Place for Mom. www.aplaceformom.com is another site for locating assisted living and nursing homes for your parent.

Visiting Angels. www.visitingangels.com this is the site to locate professional home care individuals who will tailor the type of care your parent will require according to their needs. From bathing and light housekeeping to overnight attention, these "angels" may be your answer.

Web MD. www.webmd.com is the website for WebMD. You can find information about all kinds of medical problems on this site.

ELDER CARE EQUIPMENT and CATALOGS

While some of these catalogs may have the same product, pick up a catalog from all of these companies and compare prices and specials.

If you are looking for those shelves with a railing that I mentioned in chapter 11, check out the **Geitgey's Amish Country Furnishings** on line at **www. amishcountryfurnishings.com**

Easy Comfort. This catalog has lots of cushion choices for chairs and wheelchairs, styles of walkers and devices for the walkers, items to make it easier to see, turn knobs, and do simple tasks. They have numerous articles for bathroom helpers, incontinence issues, denture products, health and beauty aids and foot products. Oh, yes, they also have the "flat" lap desk that I spoke of in chapter 11. Check out **www.easycomfort.com** If you join their Comforts Reward Club, you can save 10% on your order and greatly reduce your shipping.

Elder Depot. www.elderdepot.com has lots of things you may not have been able to find before, such as: incontinence bed pads, wheelchair cushions, bathroom safety bars, adult bibs, attractive patient gowns, a weekly pill alarm clock, photo clock . . . And they are fairly priced and offer free shipping for a minimum-sized order.

The **FeelGoodStore.com** is a great place to find some unique magnetic therapy items; supports to relieve backaches, sacroiliac pain and bad posture; and foot treatments from support shoes and creams to braces and exercise equipment. It also offers a "sound machine" called SleepMate® as mentioned in chapter 11. So check them out at: **www.feelgoodstore.com**

The catalog carrying the motto, "for Boomers and Beyond" is called **firstStreet**. They have talking wristwatches, easy-read keyboards for your computer, a hearing aid dryer and sterilizer, a variety of easy-read amplified phones, a Neptune® bath lift chair to help you in and out of the tub, Easy Climber™ chair lift on stairs, a video peephole viewer and a sleep-lift-recline chair that vibrates. Check out **www.firststreetonline.com**

Full of Life carries the slogan, "Ideas for Active Healthy Living." It truly lives up to its name as it offers help for pain relief, a variety of canes, walkers, and wheelchair devices. You'll find things that will help you reach, sit, sleep, hear and generally feel better. There is even a discreet attractive basket-weave Commode Chair that can remain in a bedroom without feeling like you're an invalid because the removable potty is hidden under the seat cushion. So check out **www.fulloflife.com**

Gold Violin offers "helpful products for **Independent Living**." They have things to help your parent in every room of their home, as well as the car. You will also find the fold-down table tray I mentioned in chapter 11. From emergency call equipment to pressure-relief wheelchair gel pads, you will be glad you checked out **www.goldviolin.com** and Gold Violin offers a 10% discount to AARP seniors.

Jitterbug®. www.jitterbug.com is the site for the senior's cell phone of choice, the Jitterbug®. It has large buttons, simple directions and even a live person to help your parent when they call the company. A cell phone can help them to stay in touch with their family and feel safer when they are on the road.

MedicAlert®. www.medicalert.com is the website for MedicAlert®. They have been around for years, making MedicAlert® bracelets. Now, they have MedicAlert® watches, sports bands, lifeline necklaces and a program called MedicAlert® Gold that keeps your parent's medical records on the internet, able to be retrieved at any time. (Just in case the internet should go down, it still helps to have a bracelet and medical information cards, like the one in this book in chapter 11.)

Sleep Solutions offers just what you might suspect and a whole lot more. There is every imaginable pillow for neck, leg, and back support, asthma suffers, side, back and tummy sleepers, sleep Apnea sufferers, as well as hair, skin and nail aids. Also, you will find a Conair® Sounds of Nature and Sleep Mate® sound machines to induce sleep, as mentioned in chapter 11 of this book. Just click on the following website **www.shopsleepsolutions.com**

Support Plus at **www.supportplus.com** is a mail order company that has everything from support stockings to ElecrtroMassage® systems. You'll find a giant variety of pillows, shoes, and a host of other helpful products in the pages of its catalog.

Whatever Works is another catalog company that has some really unique items for those who garden, still live independently and need to take care of their home, pest control or if they are just looking for ways to make life a little more pleasant safe and manageable. Check out **www.whateverworks.com**

For bird and squirrel feeders and a whole lot more: **Wild Birds Unlimited®** (stores and on line purchases at **www.wbu.com**) and **Duncraft** at **www. duncraft.com**

LEGAL STUFF

The State Bar Association will have a listing of lawyers that are in good standing. Just go to **Google.com** and type in the name of your state followed by the term, "**bar association.**" (EX: Ohio bar association)

Legal.com™ They've been around since 1991. At **www.legal.com** you will get help finding an attorney, understanding the various facets of the law in a variety of areas, be able to purchase legal forms right off your computer and in general learn a little bit about the law.

National Academy of Elder Law Attorneys can be found at **www.naela.org** After going to the site, click on ABOUT and then Facts About NAELA. Look for member directory and search the attorney in your location.

Prepaid Legal Services®, Inc. www.prepaidlegal.com is the website for Prepaid Legal Services®, Inc. For a small monthly fee, they will initially draft a will and living will for your parent and be on call for any legal questions your parent or you, as their POA on behalf of your parent, may wish to ask. They will also review any contract your parent may want to sign before they sign it. The phone questions are usually answered within 24 hours and they don't cost you anything. They will also represent your parent in court for a reduced rate. And they have an *Identity Theft Protection* plan that will notify your parent if there is any illegal activity found in the area of your parent's financial concerns, such as unusual credit card charges.

Suze Orman. www.suzeorman.com will put you in touch with Suze Orman's site. You can order her Ultimate Protection Portfolio with 50 essential documents that you can create on your computer (including the ones we covered in chapter 2).

PUPPETS

Axtell® Expressions, Inc. Professional Puppets are amazing. He has a 51" rabbit, an awesome bird illusion that looks like a comical bird perched on your arm, a duck pan and a realistic chimpanzee . . . to name a few. Check Axtell out at **www.axtell.com**

Folkmanis® Puppets are all about animals. Some of them are real looking and are great animals to go into an audience a let them pet the dog, fox, or rabbit. **www.folkmanis.com**

The Puppet Store has lots of affordable puppets for young children to work and even a portable stage, if you want to go that route. **www.thepuppetstore.com**

CDs
If you can't find these in the stores, check out Amazon.com

ANIMAL SOUNDS CDs

Since, according to the article "Heal Yourself with Animal Sounds" on Facebook, you may actually discover physical and mental health benefits by listening to or handling certain animals, I have put together a list of CDs from Amazon.com that may help your parent:

Dolphin Dreams by **Dan Gibson's Solitudes.** 2006. may actually help the body to heal.

Songbirds by the Stream by **Dan Gibson's Solitudes** may help with your parent's concentration and problem solving skills.

Echoes of Nature: Frog Chorus or **Sounds of Earth: Frogs** by **Sounds of Earth Series** may help stimulate creativity.

Sounds and Songs of the Humpback Whale by Gentle Persuasion: The **Sounds of Nature** may help induce sleep.

COMEDY CDs

Humor has often been able to lift the spirit of a depressed individual, but more recently, it has been found to help in the healing process. At the very least, comedy should make your time together more enjoyable.

Bill Cosby Wonderfulness by Bill Cosby

Something like this . . . the Bob Newhart Anthology by Bob Newhart

Emi Comedy Classics by Jack Benny

HYMNS & GOSPELS CDs

Often a senior finds it soothing to listen to spiritual music, especially when they are not able to get to church regularly or at all.

50 Golden Hymns, Vol. 1 (3 CD) (no vocal)

Blind Man Saw It All by the Booth Brothers (upbeat vocal)

Favorite Hymns with Bill and Gloria Gather (vocal included)

Gospel Music, Vol.1 by the Statler Brothers (upbeat vocal)

MUSIC & RADIO FROM THE PAST CDs

Music and other recordings from the past have actually stimulated parts of the brain that may be beneficial to a senior with dementia. Consider the following:

20th Century Masters: the Best of Bing Crosby (vocal)

The Best of the Andrews Sisters: 20th Century Masters (Millennium Collection) (vocal)

Glenn Miller Greatest Hits (instrumental)

Songs that Got Us Through WW II (vocal)

Old Time Radio All-Time Favorites (from Smithsonian Collection, a mix of comedy and more serious programming) 5 hrs.

NATURE SOUNDS

These are relaxing sounds from nature (like the sound of surf, a babbling brook or rain) that do or do not include musical instruments:

Bliss-Exceptional Nature Sounds for Relaxation, Meditation and Deep Sleep (no instruments)

Ocean Waves—Calming Sounds of the Sea (no instruments)

Dan Gibson's Solitude: Exploring Nature with Music: the Classics (includes instruments)

Dan Gibson's Solitude: Natural Stress Relief (includes instruments)

DVDs

COMEDY DVDs

As was mentioned before, under CD Comedy, humor can be a very positive tool to help relax, uplift and even heal.

Burns & Allen (George Burns and Gracie Allen)

The Golden Age of Television (**the Criterion Collection**) including Andy Griffith, Ernest Borgnine and a host of others.

Our Gang—Little Rascals Greatest Hits

Victor Borge Classic Collection (6 hours of Mr. Borge's piano classic comedy)

OLD MOVIE DVDs

The old classics can be very refreshing to a senior, especially when the TV is offering afternoon soap operas with sexual overtones and violent, often R rated movies. Here are some pleasant as well as classic musicals and dramas that should entertain most any senior.

Classic Horse Favorites: Black Beauty, the Story of Seabiscuit, National Velvet and International Velvet

Fiddler On The Rood (musical, starring Topol)

The Frank Sinatra and Gene Kelly Collection: On the Town, Anchors Away and Take Me Out to the Ball Game

It's a Wonderful Life starring James Stewart

Meet Me in Saint Louis (gentle musical of the early 1900s, starring Judy Garland)

Swiss Family Robison (whimsical adventure with an entire family stranded on an island and living in a tree house, starring John Mills)

The Sound of Music (musical of WWII era, starring Julie Andrews)

TRAVELOGUE DVDs

Whether it's a dream of someplace your parent always wanted to visit or a memory of someplace they had already been, travelogues can transport them out of their easy-chair into an entirely new setting in seconds.

Burt Wolf's Travel and Traditions: Europe Tour 6 DVDs

Reader's Digest—America's Most Scenic Drives 4 DVDs

Reader's Digest—Journey of A Lifetime 170 minutes

Do You Have a Helpful Caregiving Hint?

I'm sure you have found resource material or learned some unique ways to make the journey easier for you or the one you are caring for. If you would like to share your idea with me, just send it to: **hope@donnatrickett.com** and if I use it in my next edition of *Caregiving 101* or on my webpage, I will add a recognition statement after the idea with your name attached to it. If you include your email address, I will notify you as to where it has been posted.

Edwards Brothers Inc.
Blue Ridge Summit, PA. USA
April 13, 2011